Beating Gout

A Sufferer's Guide to Living Pain Free

Beating Gout
A Sufferer's Guide to Living Pain Free

Victor Konshin

First Edition

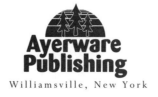

Ayerware Publishing

Williamsville, New York

Beating Gout
A Sufferer's Guide to Living Pain Free by Victor Konshin

Ayerware Publishing
Post Office Box 1098
Williamsville, NY 14231-1098
info@ayerware.com
http://www.ayerware.com
SAN: 856-1656

Edition ISBNs:
    Soft cover: 978-0-98166-244-2

First Edition, Second Printing 2008.
Printed in the United States of America

Publisher's Cataloging-in-Publication
(Provided by Quality Books, Inc.)

Konshin, Victor.
    Beating gout : a sufferer's guide to living pain free
/ Victor Konshin. -- 1st ed.
    p. cm.
    Includes index.
    LCCN 2008902977
    ISBN-13: 978-0-98166-244-2
    ISBN-10: 0-98166-244-7

    1. Gout.   I. Title.

RC629.K66 2008   616.3'999
                              QBI08-600132

Table of Contents:

Beating Gout

Introduction

For the whole of human history, people have been suffering from gout. In ancient times, only kings and noblemen could live the lifestyle that precipitated gout; but in modern times all but the poorest people in the developed world live much better than those kings and noblemen could ever have dreamed.

Today, most of us have plentiful access to nearly every kind of food the world has to offer. A trip to the grocery store is essentially a trip around the world, providing a huge variety of foods from different regions and countries. And while many of us work at jobs that may be stressful or require long hours, it is far from the backbreaking work of our ancestors. Even the nobility of past centuries would be envious of our climate-controlled offices, our modern conveniences and, most of all, our medicine.

Cases of gout were first recorded in ancient times. Yet it was only with the discovery of the drugs probenecid in 1950 and allopurinol in 1964 that gout turned from a constant menace to a condition that could be easily managed. But even now, almost 60 years later, gout is still mismanaged and mistreated.[1] I am always amazed at how often I hear stories from gout sufferers about how their doctors have been unable to find the right treatment for their condition and how they're still suffering after many years. The treatments for gout have changed very little in the past several decades, yet most doctors still have little understanding of these treatments. As a result, care varies widely.[2]

A Cautionary Tale

One sufferer, Gary, had a particularly difficult time getting his gout properly treated. It started typically, with pain and swelling in the big toe. Convinced he had an infection in his foot, Gary visited his doctor. The doctor thought it might be gout and decided an X-ray would be helpful.

When the results of the X-ray came back, the doctor immediately called Gary and told him to drop whatever he was doing and go directly to the nearest emergency room. The radiologist who examined the X-ray believed the inflammation he saw to be a potentially deadly infection of the bone called *osteomyelitis*. Gary complied, as anyone would in such a situation. He spent the next five days in the hospital, being pumped with antibiotics and subjected to a battery of tests, after which the doctors determined that Gary did, in fact, have gout.

Unfortunately, Gary's medical mistreatment didn't end there. Upon being discharged from the hospital he was given little information on what to do about his gout – other than a vague warning to stay away from seafood and beer.

Gary continued to have periodic gout attacks that frequently landed him in the emergency room. Still, none of the doctors he encountered ever explained to him the basics of gout care, much less how to properly treat the attack he was having. Even the emergency room treatment he received varied from doctor to doctor. Usually, he was sent home with prescriptions for colchicine and painkillers and told to follow up with his general practitioner.

Over time, Gary's attacks became more frequent and more severe. He asked his doctor if there was anything that could be done. The doctor prescribed a medication called allopurinol, but at the wrong dose. She never explained that in 2% of patients serious, even life-threatening side effects can occur. She also did not properly follow up on his care, nor did she prescribe the proper medication to help prevent additional attacks.

After a few weeks of treatment with allopurinol, Gary vomited violently if he drank the slightest amount of alcohol and soon noticed his skin and eyes turning yellow. Aware that these signs were not good – and were symptoms of possible liver failure – he quickly did some research and found that allopurinol can, in rare cases, cause liver toxicity. He stopped taking the drug on his own, and his liver quickly recovered.

Gary returned to his doctor and asked, "What else can I do to stop these attacks?" His doctor picked up the phone and called a pharmacist. The pharmacist suggested that the doctor prescribe colchicine, once a day. This treatment would make attacks less likely; but, as Gary later found out, is inappropriate by itself without also treating the underlying cause of gout. Gary's attacks became a little less frequent, but they still continued.

After several months of taking colchicine, Gary noticed that the big toe on his right foot had a bulge growing around one of the joints. He also started having more frequent attacks in that joint. His doctor did another X-ray and the radiologist concluded that it was harmless "soft tissue."

One day Gary felt another gout attack coming on. After experiencing dozens of attacks he could tell almost immediately that it was going to be a bad one. He immediately headed to the emergency room just as the pain went from bad to unbearable. The doctor never actually came in to see Gary, but prescribed painkillers and sent him home.

When he returned home from the emergency room, he reeled in pain all night, suffering the most intense agony he had ever experienced in his life. He took triple doses of the painkillers while downing colchicine and indomethacin (an anti-inflammatory) in dangerous quantities. He spent the next three days with severe diarrhea and vomiting frequently while his gout raged in both feet and his right knee.

The medications dulled the pain a little but this attack still lasted three full weeks. He was very lucky he did not die of an overdose or interaction from the medications he was taking. After this incident, Gary resolved to get help from an expert.

The sad truth is that Gary's tale, as bad as it was, is all too common.[1] It seems everyone I meet has a story about a friend or a relative that is still suffering from gout. It doesn't need to be that way.

So, why is gout so often mismanaged?

In 1836, English writer and clergyman Sydney Smith wrote in a letter to a friend, "I hope you and Lord Gray are well – no easy thing seeing that there are above 1,500 diseases to which Man is subject." Today, the number of diseases known to modern medicine is well above 1,500.* With such a long list of maladies, including deadly cancers and heart disease, most doctors pay little attention to "benign" ailments, such as gout.[3]

---

* To get a feel for just how many diseases are known to modern medicine go to: http://www.who.int/classifications/icd/en/. This reference lists every known disease at the time of printing and is staggeringly long.

Introduction

The second factor is that gout affects only about 1% to 2% of the general population in the developed world;* therefore, most general practitioners see only a few cases in a typical practice.[4] For these reasons, doctors often fail to keep up on the latest research, treatment methods and options.[1]

The truth, however, is that gout and its underlying disorder, hyperuricemia, are far from benign. Beyond the suffering that gout causes, hyperuricemia has been shown to be associated with a host of secondary diseases that can significantly shorten your life.[3]

One recent study found that only 22% received high-quality care for their gout and hyperuricemia.[5] This book is an effort to change that. My goal is to provide gout sufferers with the information they need to obtain the correct treatment and to make sure they do not end up living out a horror story like Gary's.

Gary eventually learned how to manage his gout and hyperuricemia. The growth on his big toe has started to shrink. And most importantly, he has not had a single gout attack since starting the course of treatment described in this book. He now knows what to do to stop a gout attack in its tracks. He still occasionally feels some discomfort, but even this is declining as his joints heal. His doctor now properly manages his gout, and he is getting the appropriate follow-up care.

This book outlines the proper treatment course and provides useful, practical information for the gout sufferer. I have left out much of the theoretical information in favor of practical information you can use to improve your health. I've also taken great pains to cite the research used in this book so that the curious reader can dig deeper into a topic if they are interested or to share it with his/her doctor.

Over 300 research papers and texts were reviewed and studied for this book; unfortunately, however, the empirical evidence in terms of the best treatment methods is weak all too often. Frequently the best information available is simply expert opinion based on years of treating gout but not backed up by scientific evidence. I have tried to indicate where the evidence is strong and where it is lacking. Fortunately, in the last five years or so, new interest by pharmaceutical companies, along with better technology, has resulted in a resurgence of research

---

* The incidence of gout has doubled over the past two decades.

into the causes and management of gout and hyperuricemia as well as its associated conditions. Also, the pace of gout research seems to be accelerating.

How to use this book

The key to beating gout is to become educated about the disease, to understand the treatments, learn how to use them and reduce the risks that this condition presents.[4] This book is designed to help you do just that, and I have worked hard to ensure that it is as accurate as possible. As with all medical advice, however, it is *not* intended to replace consultations with your regular doctor, and I cannot make ironclad guarantees that every bit of information in this book is 100% accurate and/or applicable to your individual case of gout. There are situations where the treatment of gout and hyperuricemia can be very complicated and even dangerous – this is not a do-it-yourself book.

This publication is designed to accompany the treatment from your doctor. Where your doctor's treatment differs from what this book suggests, you should politely ask why, as it is possible you have medical considerations your doctor is aware of that contradict what this book suggests. However, if you find that your doctor is not up-to-date on the latest gout treatments and research, politely refer him/her to Appendix C of this book. There, your doctor will find references to several up-to-date and very informative review articles on the latest research relating to the management of gout and hyperuricemia.

Gout and hyperuricemia can be very serious diseases. They can greatly impact your quality of life, can be crippling and are linked to many other serious conditions. Improperly treated gout may even shorten your life. There is no cure for gout, but it can and should be managed, allowing you to live a long, pain-free life. Tools that may help you achieve this goal also are available on this book's companion web site, http://www.beatinggout.com/, where updates, news and new research findings will be posted. The site allows you to leave feedback about the book and also provides a user forum where readers can exchange information and ask questions.

Chapter One:

The Four Stages of Gout

"When I have gout, I feel as if I am walking on my eyeballs"
-Sydney Smith

If gout is not treated properly it can become a crippling disease, damaging or destroying joints and resulting in constant pain along with frequent, intense and long-lasting acute attacks. Before we discuss how gout is treated, let's take a look at what causes the disease and how it progresses if untreated.

Gout is a form of arthritis, more formally known as *acute gouty arthritis* or *crystal-related arthropathy*. Unlike rheumatoid arthritis, which is caused by the immune system attacking the joint itself and eating away at it, gout is caused by uric acid crystals that form within the joints.

Why Do We Get Gout?

A long time ago – somewhere between when our ancestors were still swinging in trees and when they started to walk upright on land – something happened. Nearly every mammal on earth produces an enzyme called uricase. This enzyme's function is to degrade uric acid, the normal by-product of the metabolization of chemicals called purines.[4,6] At some point, while early humans were taking their first tentative upright steps on land, a mutation occurred in their genes, and they stopped producing uricase.[7]

This lack of uricase didn't seem to cause too much of a problem for early man. Without any form of medicine and only limited intelligence, these early bipeds survived on a sparse diet and were lucky if they made it past the age of 40. However, as man evolved further, developing bigger brains, language, agriculture and civilizations, people began living longer and with more abundance.

As their diet grew richer, their hair grayer and their lives more sedentary, nature's omission of the uricase enzyme came back to haunt them. Initially this omission only affected the wealthy - those who could afford rich foods and wine. The consumption of these rich foods (which contain higher concentrations of purines) resulted in higher levels of uric acid in their blood. Alcohol and lack of exercise made things even worse. Gout became the disease of kings and noblemen.

Over time, as the global economy and wealth grew and complex systems for transporting food products were developed, even common people became able to live with the abundance of the kings of past. Gout could strike anyone, not just the rich. Thus, gout became more common, and the portion of the population suffering from this disease continues to grow today.

Gout occurs in four stages. Not all cases progress to the final stage, but if left unmanaged, many do.

The Four Stages of Gout:

1. Asymptomatic Hyperuricemia
2. Acute Attacks
3. Intercritical Periods
4. Advanced Gout

Asymptomatic Hyperuricemia

Having high levels of uric acid in your body without experiencing any symptoms is called asymptomatic hyperuricemia. Gout will only develop in people who have had asymptomatic hyperuricemia for years or even decades.[8] Today, somewhere between 5% and 30% of people living in the developed world are hyperuricemic.[6] However, having hyperuricemia does not guarantee that you will get gout; it only predisposes you to it. About 20% of people with this condition go on to develop gout.[2,6,9]

Hyperuricemia is sometimes caused by a genetic error in the body's metabolism that causes it to produce more uric acid than normal. Or, much more commonly, it can be caused when the kidneys have difficulty removing uric acid from the body. The kidneys are very good at filtering uric acid, but about 90% of it still gets reabsorbed back into the blood before leaving the kidneys.[4] Often people can be both "over-producers" and "under-excretors" of uric acid, resulting in exceptionally high levels. This makes gout more frequent and painful, as well as more difficult to manage.

This chapter discusses the direct effects of untreated gout, but untreated hyperuricemia may pose many more health problems. There are a host of disorders associated with hyperuricemia that are much more dangerous than gout. Researchers are just starting to put the pieces of hyperuricemia and these other conditions together, and a frightening picture is developing. In Chapter Four we will discuss hyperuricemia, its causes and the diseases that scientists are now beginning to link with this condition.

Acute Attacks

Uric acid dissolves in blood serum (the liquid part of blood) and other body fluids. In people with hyperuricemia, uric acid concentrations rise to a level where it becomes a super-saturated solution,[10] meaning that more uric acid is dissolved in the body than is normally possible.

An acute gout attack occurs when these body fluids can no longer sustain this super-saturation and begin to form urate crystals; like ice crystals that form in freezing water.* These crystals can form anywhere in the body, but in a gout attack they develop in one or more of the joints.[11]

The body's immune system quickly detects these newly appearing urate crystals and assumes they are disease or infection. In response, white blood cells are sent in to attack the invaders; but when they try to devour them, the large rigid crystals burst the cells, just like popping balloons. As the white blood cells die, they release proteins telling the immune system that the cell has lost its fight with the invader and reinforcements should be sent in.

The released proteins also cause an increase in the acidity of the fluid of the joint. This makes conditions more favorable for even more urate crystals to form. The immune system responds by sending in more white blood cells and by causing

---

* Technically, urate is the salt form of uric acid. However, uric acid and urate are very often used interchangeably. For the purpose of making things as clear as possible in this book, I will refer to uric acid in a dissolved state such as in the blood as uric acid, and will call it urate when it is in a crystal form.

inflammation. More white blood cells are killed by the urate crystals, causing even more proteins to be released and more crystals to form. This process perpetuates itself, creating a runaway inflammatory response that directly causes the extreme pain of gout.[12]

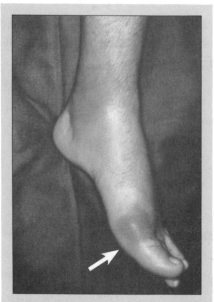

Photo 1: This photo shows the swelling and redness of podagra. ©1972-2004 American College of Rheumatology Clinical Slide Collection. Used with permission.

Most men are stricken with their first gout attack between the ages of 30-60, and most women are affected only after reaching menopause,[2,14] with gout being 5 to 8 times more common in men than women.[4] An acute gout attack typically starts with the rapid development of severe pain in the joint that reaches a peak in 6 to 12 hours. Tenderness, swelling and redness around the affected joint[18] are also typical symptoms of an attack. In severe attacks, fever and chills may also be present.[1,9,15]

A first attack of gout often occurs in the middle of the night and usually only strikes one joint. However, as the disease progresses, attacks involving multiple joints become more likely.[8,15] Eventually the inflammation process of an attack will run its course and the pain subsides on its own after a few days, but severe attacks can last weeks.[4]

The classic and very often-quoted description of an acute gout attack was written by the 17th century clinician Thomas Sydenham: "The regular gout seizes in the following manner – The patient goes to bed and sleeps quietly until about two in the morning, when he is awakened by a pain which usually seizes the great toe, but sometimes the heel, the calf of the leg or ankle. The pain resembles that of a dislocated bone… [The pain] grows gradually more violent every hour, and comes to its height toward evening [and is sometimes similar to] the gnawing of a dog and sometimes a weight and constriction of the parts affected, which become so exquisitely painful as not to endure the weight of the clothes nor the shaking of the room from a person's walking…"

Sixty percent of first gout attacks affect the second joint from the tip of the big toe. (This is known as the first *metatarsophalangeal* joint; see figure 1). An attack in this joint is also known as podagra*.[7] Gout can affect any joint in the body, but it is most common in the joints in the foot, followed by those in the ankles, hands, wrists, knees and elbows.[7,9]

Historically, gout of the hips and spine was thought to be rare, but one recent study found that gout in the spine might be frequently misdiagnosed.[16] Another interesting finding is that artificial joints are not immune to gout and can be the target of an attack.[17]

The list of reasons why asymptomatic hyperuricemia develops into gout is long; it is usually difficult to identify the exact cause in each case. Regardless, once a gout attack has occurred, additional attacks become much more likely.[3] About 60% of people who have had their first attack will have another attack within a year.[7] However, some patients do not have another attack for years after their first, while an even smaller portion never experience a second attack.[4,19]

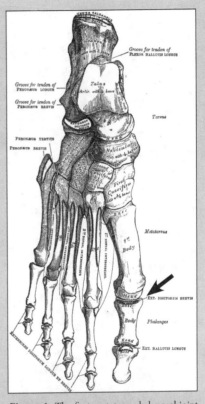

Figure 1: The first metatarsophalangeal joint of the foot (arrow) is the most common joint for early gout attacks. 60% of first gout attacks strike in this joint.

In some people with hyperuricemia, uric acid may crystallize in the soft tissues of the body and develop into what is called a tophus.[13] Tophi (plural for tophus) are masses of uric acid crystals that can form anywhere in the body, even the heart**, but most commonly appear around the joints of the arms and legs and the outer rim (helix) of the ear (See Photo 2).[9] In what is called atypical gout, tophi can occur without a person ever having a single gout attack or having experienced attacks with much more mild, diffuse pain. Atypical gout is often misdiagnosed as other forms of arthritis and is much more common in women than men.

---

* Podagra comes from the Greek word 'pous', 'pod-' that means 'foot' and 'agra' that means 'seizure.'
** Though very rare, tophi in the heart can be very dangerous.

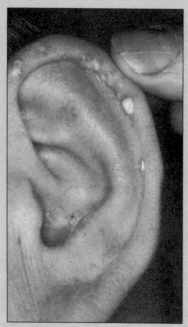

Photo 2: A photo of a person with tophi on the helixes of the ear, a common location for tophi. ©1972-2004 American College of Rheumatology Clinical Slide Collection. Used with permission.

Intercritical Periods

The time between acute attacks is known as the intercritical period.[1] The individual's uric acid levels are still high, and another attack can occur at any time. Even though there are no symptoms, damage may still be occurring. One study found that 70% of people with gout had detectable urate crystals in their joints during these intercritical periods.[18] These urate crystals are like sand in the joints, doing damage with each movement. Another study found that 25% of people reported feeling pain or discomfort during intercritical periods, lowering their quality of life.[20,21]

Over time, the frequency, duration and intensity of gout attacks usually increases. Attacks become longer and more painful, while attacks involving multiple joints become more common.[22]

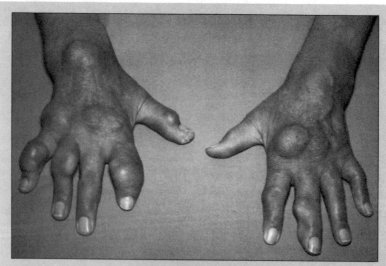

Photo 3: A photo of the hands of a person with advanced gout. Note the bulges around the joints caused by chronic swelling and tophi. ©1972-2004 American College of Rheumatology Clinical Slide Collection. Used with permission.

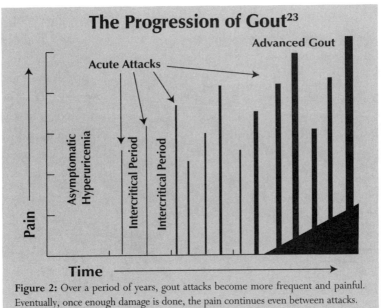

Figure 2: Over a period of years, gout attacks become more frequent and painful. Eventually, once enough damage is done, the pain continues even between attacks.

During intercritical periods, tophi may be forming. These deposits of urate crystals can grow to be very large. If tophi are close to the skin or grow large enough they may eventually break (ulcerate) or kill the skin (necrosis), allowing chalky white or yellow urate crystals to ooze out. These ulcerations may also become infected, causing additional problems.[7,9] Usually tophi form in the cooler parts of the body but they can form anywhere, even in the heart and other internal organs, potentially resulting in life-threatening conditions.

As time passes and more gout attacks occur, bony changes called "punch-out lesions" start to form around the joint. These lesions usually grow and harden over time, limiting the flexibility of the joint.[8] Eventually punch-out lesions can fuse together, totally immobilizing the joint. The presence of large tophi and punch-out lesions is sometimes called *intermediate gout*. These changes typically signal a person's progression to the last stage of gout known as advanced gout.

Advanced Gout

Advanced gout is defined as constant pain stemming from years of urate crystals degrading the joints. Joints are damaged and even destroyed completely by these crystal deposits and the accompanying constant inflammation and lesions.

Along with this come frequent, long-lasting and painful multi-joint gout attacks. Joint damage is clearly visible on X-rays, and there are usually multiple, large tophi throughout the body.[8] At this point, extensive and permanent damage has occurred and cannot be reversed. Treatment for advanced gout can only slow additional damage and reduce the occurrence of additional acute attacks.

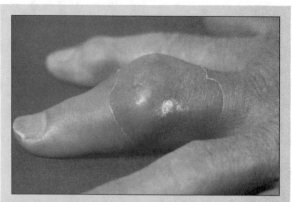

Photo 4: A photo of a patient's hand with advanced gout. The tophi growing below the skin are starting to destroy the skin above them (a condition known as skin necrosis). This skin opening can easily become infected. ©1972-2004 American College of Rheumatology Clinical Slide Collection. Used with permission.

• • •

As mentioned in the introduction, this was the normal course of the disease until 1950 and the discovery of the drug probenecid. Despite the fact that, today, gout is still often mismanaged, the good news is that gout is now a well-understood disease, and there are many tools for treating it. With a thorough understanding of how the disease progresses and what can be done to stop it, gout damage can be reversed well before it reaches the advanced stage.

If hyperuricemia is caught early and properly managed, any developing tophi can actually start to dissolve back into the blood as uric acid, where it will be removed by the kidneys.[24] Crystals that have formed in the joints also will dissolve, and the damage they caused can start to heal.[19] In the coming chapters, this book will provide you with the information you need to manage hyperuricemia, reduce or eliminate acute gout attacks, and *reverse* the progress of this disease.

As mentioned earlier, the dangers of gout do not end here. Unmanaged hyperuricemia is even more dangerous than gout itself. Chapter Four will cover the diseases associated with hyperuricemia and the dangerous health risks they pose.

Chapter Two:

Treating Gout

"Gout is the only enemy that I do not wish to have at my feet"
-Sydney Smith

As illustrated in chapter one, gout can undoubtedly be a painful and crippling disease. If left untreated or mismanaged, it can result in significant joint damage, dangerous tophi and recurrent painful attacks, all greatly affecting the gout sufferer's quality of life. Fortunately, there are medications and treatment methods that can prevent this terrible outcome. Unfortunately, however, there is little scientific evidence to confirm exactly which is the *best* gout treatment. Consequently, the "best" treatments thus are limited to the expert opinions of doctors who have been treating gout – treatments which are often contradictory. In this chapter, we will discuss the most common treatment methods, plus some recommended alternatives.

Keep in mind that this chapter describes the course of treatment for an otherwise healthy individual and will only casually refer to medical conditions that would contradict this treatment. So, please discuss this book and these suggestions with your doctor before making any changes to your current gout management and treatment. Only your doctor can make the important decisions on what medical treatments are best for your individual health.

Later chapters will discuss other actions you can take to control your gout. New research conducted in just the last few years has filled in some of the gaps in our understanding of this disease. We now have much more detailed information on the best lifestyle and dietary habits to help prevent gout as well as improve your overall health.

Treating gout can be a bit confusing at first, but once you get the hang of it, you can prevent most gout attacks from happening and stop those that do happen almost immediately.

Gout treatment consists of three parts:[9]

1. Treatment of acute gout attacks
2. Managing hyperuricemia
3. Attack prevention (prophylaxis)

Only when you understand and follow **all three parts** *can you properly control gout and minimize or eliminate gout attacks.*

Part One: Treating Acute Attacks

The key to stopping acute gout attacks is to interrupt the inflammatory process that causes the pain *before* it builds momentum. Like a runaway tractor-trailer that has lost its brakes, it's easier to stop at the top of a big hill when it is going slowest, rather than at the bottom, when the truck is traveling at high speed and totally out of control. The same is true with the runaway inflammation behind a severe gout attack. **It needs to be stopped before it builds up momentum.**[1,19]

Treating an acute attack is as simple as taking one of the medications listed below *at the very first sign of an attack.* Any delay in treating a gout attack means relief will take *much longer* to achieve. None of the doctors Gary saw ever explained this to him. So like most of us, not wanting to take medication needlessly, Gary would wait until the pain became intense before treating his attacks. He then believed the medications weren't working, when in reality he was simply taking them too late.

If you wait even a few hours, it might take days to get relief. But if you act at the very first sign of an attack, you can usually stop that attack within an hour or two – *before* the pain becomes intense. Be prepared! Keep some of this medication with you at all times! Keep some at work, in the car, next to your bed, and anywhere else where it will be readily accessible.[25] **Again, the key is to act quickly and take these medications at the very first sign of a gout attack.**[19]

Medications Used for Acute Gout Attacks

Non-Steroidal Anti-Inflammatory Medications Drugs (NSAIDs)

The medications of choice in treating acute gout attacks are called Non-Steroidal Anti-Inflammatory Drugs, or NSAIDs.[9,19,26,27] As their name implies, these medications suppress the body's inflammatory response, which is the cause of gout pain.

NSAIDs work by blocking the COX (cyclooxygenase) enzymes, which are key mediators of inflammation in the body. There are many different classes of NSAID drugs, but the ones most commonly used for gout are called *non-selective* NSAIDs. There are three different COX enzymes in the human body, and non-selective NSAIDs usually work by inhibiting the function of the first two (COX-1 and COX-2).

The other class of NSAIDs used to treat gout is called *selective* NSAIDs or *COX-2 inhibitors*. As their name implies, COX-2 drugs target only the COX-2 enzymes to prevent inflammation. In practice, these drugs have become very popular for treating gout because they typically have a lower risk of dangerous gastrointestinal side effects and appear to be as effective as non-selective NSAIDs in treating gout.[4] However, the only scientific study I found comparing a non-selective NSAID (indomethacin) and a COX-2 inhibitor drug used a COX-2 drug that is not available (etoricoxib).* This study showed this COX-2 inhibitor was just as effective as indomethacin.[28,29]

Regardless, non-selective NSAIDs are still the most commonly used medications for gout. There is a great deal of research comparing the different non-selective NSAIDs with each other as treatments for gout attacks. This research shows that all of the non-selective NSAIDs seem to be equally effective in treating attacks. Indomethacin, however, is the most commonly prescribed drug in this category, as it is one of the most powerful.[2,9]

---

* The application for etoricoxib's release to the market was recently rejected by the Food and Drug Administration which stated that the manufacturer did not provide enough evidence that the risks of this drug outweigh its benefits.

NSAIDS Used to Treat Acute Gout Attacks:

These NSAIDs have been approved by the national Food and Drug Administration (FDA) for gout and are the most commonly prescribed:[30,31]

Indomethacin

Trade names include: Apo-Indomethacin®, Indameth®, Indocid®, Indocin®, Indo-Lemmon®, Indomethagan®, Arthrexin®, Indocid® and Novo-Methacin®

Naproxen

Trade names include: Aleve®, Naprosyn®, Anaprox®, Anaprox DS®, Apo-Naproxen®, Naxen®, Novo-Naprox®, Nu-Naprox® and Naprelan®

Sulindac

Trade names include: Clinoril®, Aclin®, Apo-Sulin® and Novo-Sundac®

The COX-2 inhibiting drug most often used to treat gout is called celecoxib. Celecoxib typically has fewer gastrointestinal side effects than other NSAIDs. Yet despite its growing popularity in treating gout, celecoxib has not been approved by the FDA for this use:[32]

Celecoxib

Trade names include: Celebrex® and Celebra®

Research has shown the following NSAIDs also work well for acute gout attacks and are frequently prescribed, but again they also have not been approved by the FDA for this use:[9,30,31,33]

Ibuprofen

Trade names include: Motrin®, Advil®, Ibu-Tab 200®, Medipren®, Cap-Profen®, Tab-Profen®, Profen® and Ibuprohm®, ACT-3®, Apo-Ibuprofen®, Brufen®, Genpril®, Haltran®, IBU®, Ibu-Tabs®, Novo-Profen®, Nurifen®, Rafen® and Saleto-200®

Ketoprofen

Trade names include: Oruvail®, Orudis®, Actron®, Apo-Keto®, Novo- Keto® and Rhodis®

Piroxicam

Trade names include: Feldene®, Apo-Piroxicam® and Novo-Pirocam®

Diclofenac

Trade names include: Cataflam®, Voltaren® and Solaraze®

Note that Naproxen, Ibuprofen and Ketoprofen are available over-the-counter in the U.S. and many other countries. These medications may be good options if you feel a gout attack coming on and do not have your prescription medications with you. *However, you should discuss this option with your doctor ahead of time to make sure it's appropriate in your case.*

In addition, it is important to discuss the correct dose for these over-the-counter medications with your doctor. The dose for gout attacks (an anti-inflammatory dose) is often higher than the maximum dose printed on the label. Lastly, be sure to buy the rapid or immediate-release formula of the medication, not the sustained release.* If in doubt, ask the pharmacist.

Taking NSAIDs

Below are the *typical* doses prescribed for gout attacks. However, you should always follow the dosing that your doctor prescribes:[7,9,19,25,34]

Indomethacin:
Take an initial dose of 100 mg at the first sign of symptoms, then take another 50 mg three times a day. Stop as soon as symptoms subside; but do not take for more than two days, and do not take more than 200 mg per day.

Naproxen:
Take an initial dose of 750 mg at the first sign of symptoms, then 250 mg every eight hours. As soon as symptoms subside, reduce the dose gradually over two to three days. Do not take more than 750 mg a day after the first day, and do not take for more than 10 days.

Sulindac:
Take an initial dose of 200 mg at the first sign of symptoms then 200 mg twice a day. As soon as symptoms subside, reduce the dose gradually over two to three days. Do not take more than 400 mg a day, and do not take for more than seven days.

* In an acute gout attack it is important to stop the inflammation as soon as possible with a strong dose of NSAIDs. Sustained release formulations are designed to release a low dose over a long period of time thus it will not be strong enough to stop an attack.

Warnings About NSAIDs

NSAIDs can be dangerous if not used correctly. This applies to over-the-counter NSAIDs as well. Discuss the risks with your doctor before taking them. Be sure to read the FDA warning about these drugs in Appendix B, and always read the medication labeling or prescribing information before starting these medications. If you have questions, call your doctor and/or your pharmacist before taking them.

All NSAIDs (and indomethacin in particular) can cause dangerous gastrointestinal bleeding, ulcers and/or gastrointestinal perforation. The risk increases dramatically if you are in poor health, if you drink alcohol, take aspirin or any aspirin-containing products, take corticosteroids, or take anti-coagulants while taking NSAIDs. Gastrointestinal bleeding can happen at any time, with or without symptoms, and can be fatal.[35]

All NSAIDs can increase the risk of heart attack or stroke. This risk increases the longer you take the medication and is greater in people with preexisting heart disease. NSAID medicines should never be used right before or after a heart surgery called a "coronary artery bypass graft."[36]

Because of these dangers, NSAIDs should be used for the shortest amount of time possible. Again, taking these medications at the first sign of symptoms will minimize the length of time you will need to take them and reduce your risk of side effects.

People over age 60 or who have kidney, liver or heart problems, a history of peptic ulcers or other stomach/heartburn problems, are pregnant or are on anti-coagulants or corticosteroids, have bleeding problems or are on diuretics should not take these medications before consulting with their doctor.[9,26,33,35]

Probenecid (a uric acid-lowering medication that will be described in detail later) can reduce the rate at which some NSAIDs are removed from the body, making them more potent and potentially toxic. This also can increase the risk of dangerous side effects, including gastrointestinal bleeding. If you are taking probenecid, discuss the correct dosing of NSAIDs with your doctor *before* taking them.[35,37]

These medications may also cause allergic reactions in some people. Do not take these medications if you have ever had an allergic reaction to pain relievers, and stop taking them if you have any symptoms of an allergic reaction, such as facial swelling, hives or difficulty breathing. Call your doctor immediately. (See Appendix B for more information about NSAIDs.)

Colchicine

Colchicine has been used to treat gout for more than 2,000 years, and is still probably the most commonly prescribed medication for treating acute gout attacks. Up until the discovery of NSAIDs, colchicine was the only drug that doctors had available to treat gout.

Made from the bulb of the autumn crocus flower (scientific name: *Colchicum Autumnale*), colchicine works differently than NSAIDs. NSAIDs disrupt the function of the COX enzymes, directly limiting inflammation, whereas colchicine works by inhibiting the mobility of white blood cells.[9] If white blood cells cannot move well, they cannot effectively attack the urate crystals in the joints. This prevents the white cells from being killed by the crystals and releasing inflammation causing proteins.

I could not find any studies that directly compared colchicine to NSAIDs; however, colchicine is generally considered to be less effective in treating gout attacks than NSAIDs. Colchicine is weaker[9] and slower to act than NSAIDs.[26] It is also slow to be eliminated from the body, and as a result, it can easily build up to dangerous levels.[38]

Colchicine is a very toxic substance when taken at high doses. Its side effects include severe nausea, vomiting and diarrhea, as the body tries to rid itself of the toxin. These painful side effects obviously make colchicine an unappealing choice for treating acute gout attacks.[9]

Historically, colchicine has been used at high doses for acute gout attacks. One study found that 100% of patients who were treated with colchicine at high doses experienced these painful side effects,[39] while another found that more than 80% of patients had these symptoms before they felt relief from gout pain.[4,9] There is an old medical proverb that says "People treated with colchicine often run before they can walk."

Recently there has been substantial debate in the medical literature about using colchicine in high doses. Some experts now suggest that a lower dose can be just as effective at resolving acute attacks, while causing far fewer painful side effects.[27,40]

Regardless, colchicine should not be the first choice for acute attacks unless you have medical conditions that prevent you from using NSAIDs or you otherwise cannot tolerate NSAIDs.[39] However, colchicine is sometimes considered the better choice when the diagnosis of gout is uncertain,[19] which is perhaps one reason it is typically given by emergency room doctors instead of NSAIDs.* Colchicine can in fact play an important role in the third part of treating gout (prophylaxis), as I will explain later.

Both dosing levels are listed below, and it may require some experimentation to see which gives you the best pain relief with the least side effects. Again, as with all gout medications, the sooner you take it during an attack, the more effective it will be.[9]

Colchicine

Lower Dose Method[27]
Take .5 mg or .6 mg, three or four times a day until pain subsides or until you have taken 6 mg total. *Never take more than 6 mg for an attack.*

– or –

High Dose Method (not recommended)[25,27]
Take two 0.6 mg tablets at the first sign of attack, then one every hour until the pain subsides or nausea, vomiting or diarrhea occur. *Never take more than 6mg for an attack.*

Warnings About Colchicine

After taking a high dose of colchicine you should wait *at least* three days before taking more. As mentioned, colchicine builds up in the body, and time should be given to allow the levels to fall before taking more. Colchicine is potentially fatal

---

* Use of NSAIDs can increase the risk of gastrointestinal bleeding as well as heart attack and stroke where colchicine does not. Therefore, doctors prefer colchicine when a diagnosis is uncertain.

if more than 6 mg has been taken! If you are taking colchicine for prophylaxis (a daily dose, described in the third section), you should not use colchicine for acute attacks *at all*, as the risk of overdose is too high.

Colchicine eventually is filtered out of the body by the kidneys and liver. Kidney or liver problems increase the risk of colchicine building up to dangerous levels much more quickly, and it may therefore take longer for levels to decrease in these people. Talk to your doctor before taking colchicine if you have any kidney or liver problems.[9,38]

Also, if you have any bone marrow disease, you should discuss this with your doctor, as colchicine can suppress bone marrow. Lastly, always read the medication labeling or prescribing information, and contact your doctor *before* starting these medications if you have any questions. More information about colchicine can be found in Appendix B.

Other Medication Options for Acute Gout Attacks

If you are unable to use any of the medications discussed so far, there are additional options. Below are some other medications that are also used to treat acute gout attacks. These are usually considered second- and third-line drugs as they may carry more risks, be difficult to administer or are more expensive. Furthermore, all of these treatments are "off-label" (meaning they are not approved by the FDA) for treating acute gout attacks, even though they have been studied and are frequently used in practice.

Corticosteroids[4,7,9,25,26,27]
Corticosteroids work by suppressing the body's immune system and are some of the most powerful anti-inflammatory agents available. Injected corticosteroids can often stop attacks more quickly than other treatment options. Corticosteroids may even be the best choice for severe attacks, attacks that have gone untreated, multi-joint attacks or for people who cannot tolerate NSAIDs or colchicine.

Corticosteroids can be injected directly into the joint (intra-articular), which is usually very effective. However, this treatment is not commonly used because it must be administered by a specialist and is usually very painful. Also, in attacks involving multiple joints or the small joints of the feet or hands, a corticosteroid injection may be very difficult to administer. Lastly, there is also a risk that the medication itself may crystallize in the joint, potentially making the problem worse.

Because of these concerns, corticosteroids are usually injected into a muscle (intra-muscular). This is also highly effective, does not require a specialist, and works on both single and multi-joint attacks. Corticosteroids can also be administered through an IV.

Lastly, corticosteroids can also be taken orally, but this option is slow to act and is the least effective.

ACTH (Adrenocorticotropic hormone or corticotropin) Trade name: cortrosyn®:[9,25,32]

ACTH is a hormone secreted by the pituitary gland which has been found to be effective in treating gout attacks. However, this treatment is rarely used. Typically, it is only prescribed for people with congestive heart failure, chronic kidney failure or those who have not responded to any other treatment. It is administered by injection only.

Painkillers:[7,19,26]

Painkillers, including narcotics, are sometimes prescribed if pain is a problem. However, these medications will do little to stop the inflammation or the source of the pain, nor will they reduce uric acid levels, the source of the inflammation. Painkillers can also be highly addictive.

Rest

Another critical factor in treating gout attacks is *rest*. Remember that a gout attack is caused by needle-like crystals that form in the joint. If you start moving and stressing the joint, those crystals will act like sand, poking and grinding your joint and causing more inflammation. This increased inflammation worsens pain and could increase damage to the joint. Resting the joint for at least a day or two will result in less pain, faster recovery, and less need for medication.[9,26,41] Also, applying ice to the affected joint has been found to be helpful. (See Chapter 6.)

Summary of Part One

Stop acute attacks in their tracks by taking a NSAID, colchicine or the drug your doctor suggests *at the very first signs of symptoms.* **The key is to take the medicine as soon as possible, at the first sign of an acute attack!** Keep some of this medicine with you at all times. If you do this, you can stop the attack from turning into a character building experience in pain endurance. With quick and proper treatment, you will find that most of the time an acute attack can be stopped in an hour or two with barely a limp.

Part Two: Managing Hyperuricemia

Now that we have learned how to stop acute gout attacks, let's take a look at how to prevent them from occurring at all. Gout is caused by the buildup of uric acid (hyperuricemia) that turns into urate crystals all over the body, especially in the joints.[42] When these crystals form inside of a joint, they cause gout attacks. Since gout is caused by the build-up of uric acid, reducing the amount of this acid in the body will reduce the likelihood of attacks.[14]

In most people, hyperuricemia is a chronic, life-long condition. Consequently, people with gout will likely need to take medication for the rest of their life.[13] Only occasionally can hyperuricemia be completely managed without medications (more about this in Chapters Four and Five).

In the past, conventional wisdom said that treatment for asymptomatic hyperuricemia was unnecessary; however, many experts have started to question this. There is also much controversy on when to start uric acid-lowering treatment in people with gout.[9] Based on the research I've conducted, as well as interviews with gout experts, I feel uric acid-lowering treatments should start after the first attack and perhaps even sooner if there is a history of gout in your family, and/or you have very high uric acid levels.

However, most experts suggest waiting until after the second attack,[19] while others recommend treatment only if you have more than two or three attacks per year.[9] All, though, agree that treatment should be started immediately if tophi or joint damage has been found.[19]

As you will see later, the risk of gout increases dramatically with higher serum (blood) uric acid levels. Your doctor should check your uric acid levels a few weeks after an attack. If your serum uric acid level is found to be very high (more than 12mg/dL or 670μmol/L for men or more than 10mg/dL or 560μmol/L for women*), then uric acid-lowering treatment should probably start as soon as possible.[6] Chapter Four will describe hyperuricemia in much more detail, as well as its causes and associated conditions.

Xanthine Oxidase Inhibitor Drugs

There are two classes of drugs that can be used to treat hyperuricemia. The first is called xanthine oxidase inhibitor drugs. These medications interrupt one of the metabolic processes that creates uric acid. Currently only one xanthine oxidase inhibitor, called allopurinol, is widely available on the market.[19] Allopurinol is the drug of choice for most doctors in treating hyperuricemia. With a typical dose of just one pill per day, it is effective, has few side effects and works on people who both over-produce uric acid and under-excrete it.[2,9,19]

Allopurinol is not without risks, however; adverse reactions occur in up to 20% of patients.[19] In about 2% of patients these reactions can be very serious, and even life-threatening. If you take allopurinol and experience any adverse reactions, especially a rash, fever, yellowing of the skin or eyes, or anything that looks like an allergic reaction, contact your doctor immediately![2] Side effects that result in death are rare, but possible.

Allopurinol has potentially deadly interactions with an immunosuppressant drug called azathioprine (trade names include: Azasan®, Imuran®, Azamun® and Imurel®). This drug is used to treat organ transplant patients, for autoimmune diseases and for inflammatory bowel diseases. Allopurinol also may have deadly interactions with a drug used in leukemia patients called: mercaptopurine, 6-Mercaptopurine, 6-MP or its trade name -- Purinethol®).[24] People taking these medications should not take allopurinol.

---

* mg/dL stands for milligrams of uric acid per deciliter (100 milliliters) and μmol/L stands for micro-moles (a unit of measure) per liter. mg/dL is commonly used in the US while μmol/L is used in most other countries.

Patients who do experience mild skin rashes from allopurinol can be "desensitized" using special techniques, if the use of other uric acid-lowering drugs is not recommended.[9] However, desensitization should not be attempted if any other, more serious reaction occur. Lastly, if you have kidney problems, your doctor should watch your kidney function closely to find the correct dose for your condition.[2]

There are three additional drugs in the xanthine oxidase inhibitor class, but they are either not widely available or are in late-stage drug trials. See Appendix B for additional information on these medications.

Uricosuric Drugs

The other class of drugs used to treat hyperuricemia are called uricosuric drugs. These drugs do not stop the body from producing uric acid like allopurinol does; rather they help the kidneys filter it out.[9] Uricosuric drugs are also highly effective – some research shows them as being more effective at lowering uric acid levels than allopurinol.[2] Despite being effective, these medications are usually considered second choice drugs because of a higher risk of developing kidney stones when taking them.[43]

When taking uricosuric drugs the kidneys will remove more uric acid from the blood. This increases the concentration of uric acid in the kidneys and the urinary tract, where it may start to crystallize and form urate kidney stones. One way of preventing this is to drink at least two to three liters of water per day. This reduces the risk by lowering the concentration of uric acid in the kidneys.[9]

Another way of preventing kidney stones is to make sure your urine does not become too acidic. Urate is an acid, and urate crystals form more easily in acidic urine. Inexpensive pH test strips (also known as litmus paper), available at most drug stores and online,* can be used to monitor your urine's pH. A lower pH means your urine is more acidic.

If your urine pH is below 6, ask your doctor how you might be able to increase it. One method is to drink one or two teaspoons of baking soda in a glass of water,

---

* Look for strips that have a range of at least 5-9 in increments of at least .5 pH. Electronic pH meters are also available but are fairly expensive and more difficult to use.

up to three times a day. You may need to do some experimenting to get your urine to the optimal pH.[44] It is important to discuss this option with your doctor first, because baking soda contains high levels of sodium which can increase blood pressure.

Before starting uricosuric drugs your doctor should test how much uric acid you excrete, using a 24-hour urine test. In this test, urine is collected for 24 hours and returned to the lab to measure the amount of uric acid it contains. The 24-hour urine test will show if you are an under-excretor of uric acid or an over-producer, although it is common to be both.[45] About 90% of people are under-excretors, meaning their kidneys do not remove uric acid effectively, causing it to build up in the body.[2,4] People who over-produce uric acid and excrete it normally should not use uricosuric drugs, as they are at a much higher risk of kidney stones.[43,44]

There is significant disagreement in the medical literature about how much uric acid should be measured in a 24-hour urine test for a person to be considered an under-excretor and therefore a candidate for uricosuric drugs, but the range is *less than* 600-1,000 mg of uric acid per day.[19,33] The less uric acid you excrete per day, the less likely you are to get uric acid kidney stones when taking uricosuric drugs.[9,47] Further, if you do not produce more than 1.4 liters of urine per day you are also at higher risk for developing kidney stones.[2]

After starting uricosuric drugs, the 24-hour urine test should be performed periodically to make sure the medication is working properly and that you are not excreting uric acid at levels so high that kidney stones become a serious risk.

It's recommended that people with a history of kidney problems, kidney stones or who are over age 60 should not use uricosuric drugs*.[19] Your doctor also will want to check your kidney function before starting you on uricosuric drugs to make sure your kidneys are working properly.

Lastly, these medications affect the way some other medications work, particularly antibiotics, and they may have dangerous interactions.[43] Uricosuric drugs may affect the potency of NSAIDs and could result in them reaching toxic levels.[35] To avoid problems, make sure *all* of the doctors you are seeing are aware

---

* There is some disagreement about using these drugs in people over 60. Some experts feel that people over 60 can use uricosuric drugs as long as they have healthy kidney function.

of *all* the medications you are currently taking, including over-the-counter medicines, vitamins and herbal supplements. A more complete description of drug interactions can be found in Appendix B.

Uricosuric drugs include: Probenecid, Sulfinpyrazone (not available in the U.S.) and Benzbromarone (not available in many countries).[2] There are also drugs used for other purposes that are effective uricosuric medications, namely: micronised fenofibrate (Trade name: Tricor®) which is a cholesterol-lowering drug;[9,48] losartan (Trade name: Cozaar®) and amlodipine (Trade names: Norvasc® and Istin®) which are blood pressure-lowering drugs.[9,45,49] These medications may be an effective way to manage both conditions with one drug.[6]

Typical Uric Acid Lowering Drug Dosages:

Allopurinol: _____
   Trade names include: Lopurin®, Zyloprim®, Allorin®, Capurate® and Apo-Allopurinol®
   Start at 100 mg/day for one week; then increase to 200 mg/day for the second week, and 300 mg/day after that. Adjust dose based on serum uric acid levels. Maximum safe daily dose: 800 mg/day.[4,27]

Probenecid: _____
   Trade names include: Benemid®, Probalan® and Benuryl®
   Start at 250 mg/day increasing by 250 mg/day every two to three weeks, until 1,000 mg/day is reached (one 500 mg tablet twice a day).[43] Dosage increases are slower for this drug in order to prevent the development of kidney stones. Adjust dose based on serum uric acid levels. Maximum safe daily dose: 3,000 mg/day.[32]

Sulfinpyrazone: _____
   Trade names include: Anturane® and Anturan®
   100 mg once a day, increasing to twice a day after two to three weeks then finally to three times a day after another two to three weeks.[43] Increases are slower for this drug, again to prevent kidney stones. Adjust dose based on serum uric acid levels. Maximum safe daily dose: 400 mg/day.[27] *(Note: This medication is not available in the U.S.)*

Benzbromarone: _____

This medication has been removed from the market in many countries after being associated with fatal liver failure.[43] If this drug is available where you live, use it only as a last resort, if *all* other drugs are ineffective or contraindicated. Also, don't take this medication unless you are being closely monitored by a doctor.[1,27] Despite its risks, benzbromarone is one of the most effective uricosuric drugs available and even works in people with moderate kidney failure.[2,43] See Appendix B for information on other medication options.

Using Uric Acid Lowering Medications

Lowering uric acid levels will reduce the risk of gout attacks. However, it has been shown that fluctuations in blood uric acid levels can actually bring on gout attacks. Therefore it's important to avoid any major fluctuation in your uric acid levels.

When Starting Uric Acid Lowering Treatment

1. **Do not start taking uric acid-lowering medications during or shortly after a gout attack.**[1,9] Attacks cause blood levels of uric acid to fluctuate. Starting uric acid-lowering treatment at this time will make levels fluctuate even more, increasing the chances that you will have another attack or making your current attack worse.[2,19] Wait at least two to three weeks (some doctors suggest six to eight weeks) after an attack to allow your uric acid levels to settle.

    If you do have an attack while taking any of these uric acid-lowering medications, *do not stop taking them!*[26] Remember, fluctuations in your uric acid levels will make things worse, which is what will happen if you stop taking these medications or change the dosage level during an attack.[1,26]

2. **Start at a low dose.** Regardless of which uric acid-lowering medication you take, it needs to be started at a low dose and built up to the full dose over several weeks.[4,19]

3. **Stick with it.** Starting uric acid-lowering treatment will not stop attacks immediately; in fact, it may *increase* them.[2] If you have an attack while taking one of these medications, don't be discouraged. It may take a while, as long as six months to a year, to lower uric acid levels to the point where the attacks stop.[13] Remember, hyperuricemia means high uric acid levels *everywhere* in the body, not just the blood. It will take time for uric acid levels throughout your body to stabilize.

One of the biggest problems with treating gout is patient compliance.[2] People start taking the medications, have more attacks, and figure they just don't work. They are working! Stick with it! Treat acute attacks as described in the previous section. The next part of gout treatment, called prophylaxis and will help prevent these attacks.

Follow-Up

Unfortunately, General Practitioners have not done well providing follow-up for people on uric acid-lowering medications. *During the first three to six months after you start these medications, your Doctor should check your serum uric acid levels every two weeks to four weeks and adjust the dosages to maintain target levels.*[9,19,42] As someone with gout, you should know your uric acid level just as people with diabetes know their blood sugar level. It is *your* health, and you should play an active role in your own well being and treatment.

Most experts consider the target of uric acid-lowering treatments to be a blood serum uric acid level of ***less than*** 6mg/dL (360μmol/L).[4,9,19,27] But new guidelines set by the British Society for Rheumatology suggest an even lower level of ***less than*** 5mg/dL (278μmol/L).[42] There is no scientific evidence on what the best level is, but it is generally agreed that the lower the better.[13] Once uric acid levels have *stabilized* under this level, experts suggest testing should be done annually, and dosing adjusted to stay below the target level. However, blood uric acid levels can vary significantly during the day, so more frequent testing might be needed. Unfortunately, there is no research yet to determine the best testing schedule.[42]

Some experts are now suggesting that a combination of xanthine oxidase inhibitor drugs (allopurinol) and uricosuric drugs (probenecid) may be most effective in people with very high uric acid levels or in those for whom single drug therapy alone does not lower acid levels to the target range.[50] This may also be the best course of treatment for people who both over-produce and under-excrete uric acid.

Again, *always* read the medication labeling or prescribing information and contact your doctor *before* starting these medications if you have any questions. And make sure to ask your doctor about what medications you can safely take in combination if an attack occurs.

Summary of Part Two

To manage hyperuricemia, the underlying cause of gout, start uric acid-lowering treatment two to three weeks after your last attack, and stick with it! This will lower your blood uric acid levels so that further attacks are far less likely. Start at a low dose, and work your way up over time. Do not start or stop taking this medication or change dosage amounts during an attack.

Remember, it will take a while for uric acid-lowering treatments to stop attacks. It may take a year or more if you have had many attacks in the past or if you have tophi. *Stick with it, and it will work!*

Part Three: Prophylaxis

Uric acid-lowering treatments lower blood levels of uric acid, making it possible for uric acid in other body tissues to dissolve into the blood and be removed. This process can cause uric acid levels to fluctuate and can increase the frequency of gout attacks.[2]

Fortunately, acute attacks can be prevented with the use of prophylaxis.[9,19,25] Simply put, prophylaxis is taking a low dose of one of the drugs used to treat acute attacks in order to prevent an attack from ever getting started. You should only use prophylactic treatment if you are also taking uric acid-lowering medications.[19]

The most commonly used drug for prophylaxis is colchicine. As said earlier, colchicine can cause significant side effects at doses high enough to treat acute attacks; but most patients experience few, if any, side effects at the much lower prophylaxis dose. Since colchicine does not cause the dangerous side effects that NSAIDs do, it is also much safer than NSAIDs when taken long-term.[2,27] However, if you cannot take colchicine for whatever reason, low-dose NSAIDs may also be an option.

Prophylactic treatment is meant to be temporary, to reduce the number and intensity of attacks until the uric acid-lowering treatment can do its job. However, there is significant disagreement on the dose and length of time of prophylactic treatment.[2] Some experts suggest only three months are needed, while others suggest at least a year. Still others have suggested that prophylaxis should be maintained until the patient's blood uric acid levels have stabilized in the normal range (*less than* 6mg/dL or 360μmol/L), all tophi have dissolved, *and* you have not had a gout attack for three to six months. Unfortunately, little scientific evidence is available on the best length of time for prophylactic treatment, just expert opinion.[9,19,49]

The length of time you will need to use prophylaxis may depend on how many previous attacks you have had. Research has shown that the more attacks you have had, the more likely you are to have more. Therefore, the more attacks you have had, the longer you may need to be on prophylaxis.[13] It might be best to try to wean yourself off prophylaxis after three months. If you start to experience symptoms or have an attack, start it back up again for another three months, then try again to wean yourself off.

Many of the medications mentioned so far can interact with each other, so again, it's important to discuss these interactions with your doctor.[25]

Prophylaxis Dosing:
Colchicine: 0.5mg - 1.8mg a day.[25]
— or —
Indomethacin: 25mg twice a day for up to six months.[19]
— or —
Naproxen: 250mg per day.[2]

Important note: If you take colchicine for prophylaxis, you should *not* take colchicine to treat acute attacks, as the risk of overdose is very high. Whenever you are in doubt, it's best to check with your doctor.

Summary of Part Three

When beginning uric acid-lowering treatment, also start on prophylactic treatment to lower the risk of an attack. Low-dose colchicine, indomethacin or naproxen are the most common medications for this. Stick with it for at least three months before trying to wean yourself off, but be aware that it may take a year or longer. Also, do not stop taking this medication during an attack.

An Alternative Treatment Method

Experts in the field of gout have reviewed this book prior to publication. One expert with more than 45 years of clinical experience has developed his own method of treating gout over the years.

He believes that acute attacks are best treated with multiple drugs taken simultaneously. He also feels that uric acid lowering treatments should be started during the very first gout attack (not waiting several weeks) and at a very low dose, increasing it very gradually.

Alternative Treatment for Gout Attacks:

1. **Use low-dose colchicine:** Take .6 mg of colchicine up to four times a day until symptoms subside or you have taken 6 mg.
2. **At the same time, take an NSAID** that your doctor feels is best, given your medical condition and history.
3. **Receive an inter-muscular injection of a corticosteroid** such as methylprednisolone (Trade name: DepoMedrol®) as soon as is practical. Corticosteroids are powerful anti-inflammatory medications but must be injected to be most effective.

4. **If needed, pain medications** such as dextropropoxyphene (Trade names: Darvocet N®, Balacet®, Capadex®, Paradex® or Di-Gesic®) or Tylenol® (acetaminophen, also known as paracetamol) with codeine can be used.

5. **If you are not already taking a uric acid-lowering medication, start immediately at a very low dose.** He suggests not waiting two to three weeks as recommended above, but rather starting immediately at a very low dose and increasing the dose very slowly to full strength to maintain the target uric acid level (under 6mg/dL or 360μmol/L). This treatment should start at the very first gout attack and be maintained for life, unless a secondary cause for the hyperuricemia can be found. (See Chapter Four.)

This expert also believes that prophylaxis is unnecessary if uric acid-lowering treatment is started with the very first attack. Additionally, he feels that not treating asymptomatic hyperuricemia is often a mistake. He noted that in his own practice, he has recently seen an explosion in the number of people with large tophi and believes that this is the result of the failure to treat asymptomatic hyperuricemia.

This may also be the result of allopurinol use. Allopurinol lowers uric acid levels by reducing the production of uric acid, but in people who also do not excrete enough uric acid, this may not be enough. It might be effective at stopping attacks but not at preventing tophi from forming. Therefore, he recommends the addition of a uricosuric drug such as probenecid (along with allopurinol) may be needed in some cases.

Three Parts of

Part 1: Stopping a Gout Attack

Key: The key is to stop the inflammation response of an attack as soon as possible. Start treatment at the very first sign of an attack. Waiting even a couple of hours will result in a much longer and more painful attack.

Medications:

Most commonly used NSAIDs:
Indomethacin, Naproxen or Sulindac

Cox-2 Inhibitors:
Celecoxib

Part 2: Managing Hyperuricemia

Key: Hyperuricemia (high uric acid levels) causes gout. These medications work by lowering uric acid levels. The goal of treatment is to lower serum uric acid levels to less than 6mg/dL or $360\mu mol/L$.

Medications:

Reduces uric acid production: Allopurinol

Increases uric acid excretion: Probenecid and Sulfinpyrazone

Important Points (all medications):
- Wait two to three weeks after an attack before beginning treatment.
- Start at a low dose and gradually increase.
- Watch for potentially dangerous side effects.
- Do not stop taking these medications if an attack occurs.
- Use prophylactic treatment to reduce the chance of an attack.
- Monitor your uric acid levels frequently at first, then annually.

Part 3: Prophylaxis

Key: When starting uric acid-lowering treatment, attacks can increase. Prophylaxis is used to reduce the frequency and intensity of attacks. Use for at least three months, but be prepared to stay with it for up to a year.

Preferred: Low-dose Colchicine

Alternative Options: Low-dose Indomethacin or Naproxen

Gout Management

Other NSAIDs:

Ibuprofen, Ketoprofen, Piroxicam or Diclofenac

Alternative Options or Complimentary Medications:

Colchicine, Corticosteroids or ACTH

Only take medications and doses prescribed by your doctor. Keep some medication with you at all times. Read all warnings, and discuss the risks with your doctor before taking any medication. Stop using medications as soon as symptoms subside.

Important Points (Probenecid and Sulfinpyrazone):
- A 24-hour urine test should be done before starting.
- Over-producers of uric acid should not take these medications.
- Drink at least two to three liters of water per day.
- Test urine pH regularly. If under 6, discuss with your doctor.

Other Medication Options:
- Micronised fenofibrate if you have high cholesterol.
- Losartan or amlodipine if you have high blood pressure.

Always take only the exact medications and doses prescribed by your doctor. Read all warnings, and discuss the risks with your doctor before taking any medication.

Always take only medications and doses prescribed by your doctor. Discuss the correct medications to take in the case of acute attack with your doctor. Read all warnings and discuss risks with your doctor before taking any medication.

Chapter Three:

Getting the Right Diagnosis

"The best medicine I know for rheumatism is to
thank the Lord that it ain't gout."
-Josh Billings

One of the most critical components of gout treatment is getting an accurate diagnosis.[2] There are several conditions that look like gout, and some are very serious, even life-threatening, so it is critical that you first get a definitive diagnosis.[4] Getting an accurate diagnosis for gout sounds straightforward, but misdiagnosis is much more common than you would think as gout can be easily confused with several other conditions.

The most dangerous condition that can look like gout is called septic arthritis, which is an infection of the joint.[51] Though rare, this is a very serious condition with an 11% fatality rate.[18] Because gout attacks can occur with chills and fever, just as an infection would, and because septic arthritis and gout occasionally occur at the same time,[7,51] it is important to make sure there is no infection.

Synovial Fluid Diagnosis

The most accurate test for diagnosing gout is to directly test the fluid inside the joint for urate crystals and infection. To do this, the doctor will use a fine needle to extract fluid directly from a joint during an attack.[2] This fluid, called synovial fluid, is examined under a microscope to look for tell-tale needle-shaped urate crystals. Using polarized light, urate crystals appear with a specific color and shape, making them easy to differentiate from other types of crystals that can form in the joints. (We will discuss those later.)[2,8,52]

To test the synovial fluid for infection (septic arthritis), the fluid is placed into a Petri dish, then into an incubator to see if any bacteria grow. This test is known as a "culture." A culture, along with a white blood cell count of the fluid, will

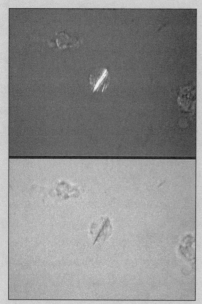

Photo 1: A photo of a urate crystal stuck through a white blood cell like a toothpick through a martini olive. This is the result of the white blood cell trying to ingest it but it ends up killing the cell and causing the inflammatory response of gout. The top half of the image is what is seen through polarized light – the urate crystal "lights up." ©1972-2004 American College of Rheumatology Clinical Slide Collection. Used with permission.

show if infection is present.[7] Once a diagnosis of gout has been confirmed and infection is ruled out, there is usually no need to undergo this test again.

Though it sounds unpleasant to have a needle poked into a joint during an attack, most people handle it quite well. The test is well worth enduring to get a definitive diagnosis of gout and to ensure there is no infection. With this diagnosis, treatment can proceed with confidence.[2]

Synovial fluid tests are definitive for diagnosing gout if uric acid crystals are present, but uric acid crystals are seen only 84% of the time. This means that 16% of the time, the person examining the sample misses the tell-tale crystals, or the crystals have dissolved back into the fluid while under the microscope.[7] If your doctor suspects gout but the synovial fluid test is negative, the test might need to be redone.[2]

Tophi Sampling Diagnosis

Another way of getting a definitive diagnosis applies to cases where the presence of tophi is suspected. A sample of the substance inside the tophi is extracted with a needle and analyzed. If this sample contains urate crystals, then gout can be definitively diagnosed, although this does not rule out the possibility of septic arthritis.[53]

Analysis of synovial fluid is the most accurate diagnosis, but it is not commonly performed. This is because it usually requires a specialist to extract the synovial fluid, and that fluid must be analyzed immediately. Also, sampling tophi is uncommon, because tophi are usually not present in early-stage cases of gout. Usually the diagnosis is built based on its clinical features.[18,42]

Clinical Diagnosis

Known as the Wallace Criteria, after the doctor that first developed them in 1977, gout can be diagnosed if six of the symptoms below are present. This is currently one of the most commonly used methods for diagnosing gout:[7,53]

- Uneven swelling within a joint on an x-ray.
- First metatarsophalangeal joint (second joint from the tip of the big toe) is tender or swollen (i.e., Podagra).
- Hyperuricemia is confirmed using a blood test.
  (Note: uric acid levels are often normal during an attack)
- Severe inflammation developed within one day.
- Attack affects only a single joint.
- More than one acute arthritis (gout) attack.
- Redness observed over affected joint(s).
- Subcortical cysts without joint erosions on an x-ray.
  (These are changes seen on an X-ray during an attack.)
- The patient has suspected tophi.
- There is an attack in only the second joint from the tip of the big toe (known as the first metatarsophalangeal joint.)
- There is an attack in only one joint in either the ankle or upper foot.
- The joint fluid culture is negative for infection during an attack.

Blood Tests

Blood tests do not play a role in the diagnosis of gout other than to establish the presence of hyperuricemia. As mentioned earlier, 80% of people with hyperuricemia never get gout; therefore a high serum uric acid level (sUA) might simply be the result of asymptomatic hyperuricemia, while the symptoms could be due to another condition.[2,18,54]

Furthermore, during an acute attack sUA levels measure in the normal range about 60% of the time. This is likely due to uric acid being used up to form urate crystals, pulling uric acid out of the blood.[4,52] Thus, the role of blood tests in the diagnosis of gout is fairly small.

Nonetheless, sUA level blood tests do play an important role in the long-term management of gout.[15] These tests are used to confirm the effectiveness of uric acid-lowering treatments and to adjust dosing of medication.[9,42] Remember that the goal of uric acid lowering treatment is to bring levels down *below at least* 6mg/dL (333μmol/L). The sUA blood test is used to verify that these target levels have been reached.

Lab test reports sometimes show sUA levels as high as 8.5mg/dL (472μmol/L) as being "normal."[13] This is because the normal range shown on these reports is derived from averaging the results of all the other patients tested by that lab. Since up to 30% of the public may be hyperuricemic, this skews the "normal" range upward. If your doctor says your level is normal, ask him or her exactly what your sUA level is. If it is above 6mg/dL (333μmol/L), discuss ways to bring it down even further. (See Chapter Five.) As someone with hyperuricemia and gout, you should know your sUA level, just as someone with diabetes knows their blood sugar level.

Urine Tests

There are no urine tests used in diagnosing gout. However, a 24-hour urine test can help to determine whether your body excretes uric acid normally or not. If you over-produce uric acid and excrete it at normal levels, then using uricosuric drugs such as probenecid will increase uric acid excretion further and result in a higher risk of urate crystals forming kidney stones. However, if allopurinol is used, this test may be unnecessary, since allopurinol *reduces* the production of uric acid and does not increase excretion. Therefore this test is usually only done if you cannot take allopurinol and your doctor is considering putting you on a uricosuric drug.[2] (See Chapter Two.)

Diagnostic Imaging

Currently, there are no diagnostic imaging techniques that can replace synovial fluid analysis[55] or otherwise provide a definitive diagnosis for gout. However, several techniques can provide limited evidence in forming a diagnosis or for evaluating damage caused by the disease.

X-Ray Tests:

X-ray tests can provide some useful information in diagnosing gout. Early stages show uneven swelling in soft tissues around affected joints, which are fairly specific to gout.[8] (These are about 90% accurate.) However, this swelling shows up only about 42% of the time.[7]

X-rays are useful in cases where gout has gone undiagnosed and untreated for a long time. X-rays can show the extent of joint damage but this damage can be easily confused with damage caused by other conditions, such as rheumatoid arthritis.[4,18,56] Also, tophi and urate kidney stones are transparent to X-rays and cannot be seen directly, again limiting the usefulness of X-rays.

High-Resolution Ultrasound:

High-resolution ultrasound is one of the newest diagnostic techniques for gout. It has not been well studied,[46] and it is also not widely available, but it is becoming a useful tool in providing diagnostic information.[57,58] In addition, high-resolution ultrasound can be used to evaluate any joint damage resulting from uncontrolled disease.[59] It's unlikely that ultrasound will ever provide a definitive diagnosis by itself, but it can be a useful tool in identifying gout.[58]

CT and MRI scans:

These scans are not typically used for gout, except in cases of advanced gout where extensive joint damage has already occurred. CT and MRI scans may someday prove to be useful in gout diagnosis, but they have not yet been studied, and no procedures exist for this purpose.[2,8,55]

Nuclear Medicine (bone scans):

Bone scans can be useful in measuring the extent of damage caused by gout and can help in building a diagnosis, but they are usually only performed when other techniques are difficult or impossible.[60]

Other Conditions That Look Like Gout

Here is a list of many (but not all) conditions that may look like gout.[4,61] Your doctor should try to eliminate the most dangerous of these conditions before gout is positively diagnosed, and the other possibilities should be considered if the standard treatments outlined in this book are not effective.

Septic (Infectious) Arthritis:

A very serious condition with an 11% fatality rate. It can be caused by various bacterial and fungal infections and should always be ruled out when diagnosing gout.

Other Types of Crystal-Induced Arthritis:

Pseudogout: This has very similar symptoms as gout, except it's caused by calcium pyrophosphate crystals, rather than uric acid crystals.[2]

Hydroxyapatite Arthritis: Hydroxyapatite is a major component of normal bone and teeth. Hydroxyapatite crystals are too small to be seen under a standard microscope and require an electron microscope to be identified.[62]

Calcium Oxalate Arthritis: This condition is also very similar to gout, except it is caused by calcium oxalate crystals rather than uric acid crystals. Typically this disease affects patients on kidney dialysis.

Rheumatic Arthritis:

Rheumatic Arthritis: RA is what most people usually think of as arthritis, and is caused by the body's immune system attacking joint tissues. It generally affects multiple joints simultaneously, but is sometimes mistaken for gout.[63]

Rheumatic Fever: May develop after certain streptococcal infections, such as strep throat or scarlet fever.

Psoriatic arthritis: Arthritis that is caused by psoriasis.[64]

Seronegative Spondyloarthropathies: A series of genetic inflammatory joint diseases.

Intermittent Rheumatisms: Among these are palindromic rheumatism, hydrarthrosis, familial Mediterranean fever, Behcet's disease and reactive arthritis.

Systemic Lupus Erythematosus and Other Connective Tissue Diseases: These include scleroderma, mixed connective tissue disease, polymyositis/dermatomyositis and relapsing polychronditis.

Vasculitis: Inflammation of the walls of blood vessels.

Adult Still's Disease: A rare rheumatic disorder that is usually accompanied by a fever.

Other Conditions:

Amyloidosis: A protein disorder.

Sarcoidosis: An immune system disorder.

Certain Acute Leukemia and Lymphomas: Certain types of cancer

Paraneoplastic Arthritis: A reaction caused by cancer in another part of the body.

Diseases that deposit substances throughout the body: Includes ochronosis, hemochromatosis, Wilson's disease and hyperlipemias.

Posttramatic Arthritis: Arthritis that results from a traumatic injury.

Chapter Four:

Hyperuricemia

"Once gouty, always gouty"
-Medical Proverb

Hyperuricemia is the underlying cause of gout. Therefore, understanding hyperuricemia is a critical concern for gout sufferers. While not everyone with hyperuricemia will develop gout, hyperuricemia is associated with other dangerous and debilitating conditions that can seriously affect quality of life.

What is Hyperuricemia?

Hyperuricemia means too much uric acid in the body. Uric acid is a normal by-product of several types of metabolic processes. In most people, there is a balance between the rate at which uric acid is created and the rate at which it's removed from the body. In people with hyperuricemia, however, this system is out of balance. In practice, hyperuricemia is defined as a blood serum uric acid level of over 7mg/dL (389μmol/L) in men and 6.5mg/dL (361μmol/L) in post-menopausal women.[65]

Approximately 90% of people who are hyperuricemic *produce normal* amounts of uric acid but have *problems eliminating it* from their bodies. The other 10% *produce too much* uric acid. Interestingly, however, it is not uncommon to *both* under-excrete and over-produce uric acid.

About two-thirds of uric acid is removed from the body by the kidneys, while the other third is removed through the intestines. Since there is no way to control how much uric acid is removed from the body through the intestines, treatments focus on helping the kidneys remove excess uric acid or else interfere with the production of uric acid.

However, those with hyperuricemia have high levels of uric acid throughout their body, not just the blood. This is why uric acid-lowering treatments may take so long to control gout attacks – it takes time to remove excess uric acid from *all* areas of the body, for it to be dissolved in the blood, and then removed by the kidneys.

Why Does Hyperuricemia Occur?

In men, uric acid levels typically begin to increase after puberty and usually continues to climb throughout life.[9] For women, estrogen plays an important role in the control of uric acid, which is why it's rare for women to have hyperuricemia or gout before menopause. After menopause, the incidence of hyperuricemia in women increases, but is still only about a third of that of men.[14] Nevertheless, there is a rare condition in which pregnant women can develop hyperuricemia and gout.[33]

About 90% of hyperuricemia cases are known as *idiopathic*, meaning the exact cause is unknown. These are likely due to a genetic error in the body's metabolic systems that causes increased production of uric acid and/or genetic factors that reduce the body's ability to remove uric acid. When gout results from idiopathic hyperuricemia, these cases are called "primary gout." Primary gout *cannot* be cured, only managed.[8]

Since primary gout is often genetic, it usually runs in families. The likelihood of a family member of a gout sufferer developing gout is between 6-80%*,[8] compared to only 1% for those who do not have a family member with the disease. Also, both men and women with a strong genetic predisposition to gout will tend to get gout earlier in life.[69]

People of Pacific Island descent also have a much higher incidence of hyperuricemia and gout than those of other ethnic groups. Pacific Islanders have genetic differences that cause them to develop severe hyperuricemia when they consume a Western-style diet.[8,71] African Americans are also at a somewhat higher risk, but the reason is not yet well understood.[70]

---

* This very wide range is due to the fact that some ethnic groups, such as Pacific Islanders, are much more susceptible to gout than other groups. I could not find statistics that break this down further.

For the other 10% of people who are hyperuricemic, it is caused by another underlying medical condition. If it results in gout, this is known as "secondary gout."[11] Doctors should look for a secondary cause of hyperuricemia whenever gout is diagnosed, as some of these secondary causes can be very serious.[4,13,19] It is possible for people with primary gout to have a secondary condition that makes their hyperuricemia worse.

Some Causes of Secondary Gout[2,4,9,65]

- Nutrition, alcohol, obesity and lifestyle are the most common causes of secondary gout. They also are often found in people with primary gout, worsening their the condition. (These issues will be addressed in the next chapter.)
- Metabolic syndrome (described later in this chapter)
- Kidney problems
- Severe psoriasis
- Hypertriglyceridaemia (high levels of triglycerides in the blood)
- Myeloproliferative diseases (diseases of the bone marrow)
- Lymphoproliferative diseases (diseases where too many white blood cells are produced) including cancers of the blood or bone marrow.
- Chemotherapy
- Hypertension (high blood pressure)
- Medications including:
  - Ciclosporin or cyclosporine (prescribed for transplant patients and people with psoriasis)
  - Diuretics including, but not limited to,*:[14]
    - Thiazides (drugs used for high blood pressure, also known as "loop diuretics")
    - Furosemide or frusemide (used to treat heart failure)
  - Ethambutol or myambutol (used to treat tuberculosis)
  - Pyrazinamide (used to treat tuberculosis)
  - Low-dose aspirin (See Chapter Five.)
  - Levodopa (used to treat Parkinson's disease)
  - Niacin (more commonly known as vitamin B_3)

* Diuretic use is one of the most common causes of secondary gout, particularly in post-menopausal women.

- Metabolic/hormonal abnormalities including:
  - Lactic acidosis (build-up of lactic acid in the blood)
  - Ketosis (liver problems)
  - Hypothyroidism (under-active thyroid gland)
  - Hyperparathyroidism (over-active parathyroid gland)
  - Lesch–Nyhan syndrome
  - Von Gierke's disease
- Lead poisoning
- Fructose intolerance
- Post-operative dehydration or starvation
- Sleep-associated hypoxemia (sleep problems that result in oxygen deprivation)[72]
- Sarcoidosis (an immune system disorder)
- Toxemia of pregnancy (pre-eclampsia)
- Sickle cell disease
- Down's syndrome
- Myogenic diseases
- Phosphoribosyl pyrophosphate synthetase super-activity (a genetic disorder)
- Infantile autism
- HIV infection[19]
- Laxative abuse as in anorexia nervosa[19]

Gout typically appears only after years or even decades of uncontrolled hyperuricemia, which is why most cases develop in people over the age of 40.[8] Cases of gout in people under 30 are possible, but rare, and are usually due to a secondary cause.[2,6]

The degree of hyperuricemia directly affects your likelihood of developing gout,[2] as well as the frequency with which your gout attacks occur (see figure 1).[66,67,68] The higher your uric acid level, the more likely it is you will have gout, and the attacks will be more frequent. Therefore, the goal of gout treatment is not to reduce attacks, but to lower uric acid levels and thus prevent attacks.[27]

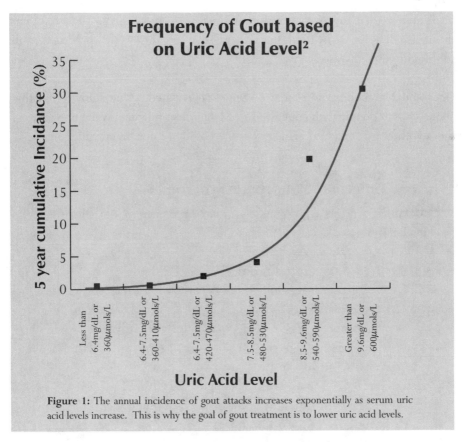

Figure 1: The annual incidence of gout attacks increases exponentially as serum uric acid levels increase. This is why the goal of gout treatment is to lower uric acid levels.

Conditions Associated with Hyperuricemia and Gout:

Hyperuricemia and gout have been linked with several very serious diseases.[6] Scientists are now just starting to look at how these conditions are related to one another and cannot yet say that hyperuricemia or gout *causes* any of them.[19,73] What can be said is that in people with hyperuricemia and gout, these other conditions are often also present. A diagnosis of gout should be a red flag for your doctor to look for these associated conditions, as they can be very serious.[18,19,27,70,74,75]

Metabolic Syndrome (also known as Syndrome X, insulin resistance syndrome, Reaven's syndrome or CHAOS): Metabolic syndrome is a combination of disorders that, when put together, greatly increase your likelihood of developing several very deadly diseases, including: cardiovascular disease and heart attacks, diabetes, stroke and numerous types of cancer.[75] Metabolic syndrome is not a disease by itself, but rather a set of conditions that predispose you to this cluster of diseases.

Gout and Metabolic syndrome are strongly correlated. One study found that about 75% of people with gout also had Metabolic syndrome, while only 25% of those without gout had it.[4] This risk was even higher in women with gout.[75]

Conditions of the Metabolic Syndrome:

Metabolic syndrome is defined as having three or more of the following conditions:[76,77]

Elevated waist circumference:
> Men – A waist circumference equal to or greater than
>> 40 inches (102 cm)
> Women – A measurement equal to or greater than
>> 35 inches (88 cm)

Elevated triglycerides:
> Equal to or greater than 150mg/dL (170μmol/L)
> or are on drug treatment for elevated triglycerides

Reduced HDL ("good") cholesterol:
> Men – Less than 40mg/dL (90μmol/L)
> Women – Less than 50mg/dL (110μmol/L)
> or are on drug treatment for reduced HDL-C

Elevated blood pressure:
> Equal to or greater than 130/85
> or are on antihypertensive drug treatment and have a
> history of hypertension

Elevated fasting glucose:
> Equal to or greater than 100mg/dL (560μmol/L)
> or are on drug treatment for elevated glucose

People with Metabolic syndrome are nearly three times more likely to develop atherosclerosis (blockage of the arteries) and are up to five times more likely to develop Type 2 diabetes. Metabolic syndrome also increases your likelihood of dying from all causes, cardiovascular disease in particular.[2,75]

Hyperuricemia has also been suggested as an independent symptom of insulin resistance, the precursor to diabetes. People who also have hyperlipidemia (high lipid levels) may be at a higher risk for insulin resistance-related cardiovascular diseases, particularly individuals who carry extra pounds around their abdominal area.[78]

Heart Disease: Even without Metabolic syndrome, hyperuricemia has been shown to be strongly associated with cardiovascular disease.[79] Hyperuricemia is a strong risk factor for coronary heart disease, peripheral artery disease, congestive heart failure, vascular (blood vessel) diseases such as atherosclerosis, and death from all other cardiovascular diseases.[6,7,80,81] These risks increase even further for people who also have high blood pressure.[78]

One research study found that for each 1mg/dL (59μmol/L) increase in blood serum uric acid levels, a person's risk of death from cardiovascular disease increases by 9% and their risk of dying from coronary heart disease increases by 17%. The biggest jump in cardiovascular disease deaths occurred in patients with uric acid levels above 5.2mg/dL (310μmol/L), and it is believed that the risk increases rapidly at higher uric acid levels.[79] Another large study showed that the risk of coronary artery disease in people with hyperuricemia is about 60% greater than those without it.[82]

The scientific literature shows that the risk of heart disease due to hyperuricemia is high enough to rank it third behind smoking and a family history of heart attacks. Also, the risk is higher in women than in men.

High Blood Pressure: Hyperuricemia is also a predictor of high blood pressure. Forty-four percent of people with hyperuricemia and gout also have high blood pressure.[2] One research study found that for every 1mg/dL (56μmol/L) increase in serum uric acid levels there is a 23% increase in the risk of high blood pressure. It has also been linked to stroke, pulmonary arterial hypertension (high blood pressure in the artery connecting the heart and the lungs), and pregnancy-induced hypertension (pre-eclampsia). Additionally, there appears to be a connection between high blood pressure and hyperuricemia that results in kidney damage.[6] Lastly, diuretics used to treat high blood pressure can significantly increase uric acid levels.[70]

Kidney Disease: There is also a very strong link between hyperuricemia and chronic kidney disease.[6,78] One large study from Japan found that people with high uric acid levels (over 8.5mg/dL or 470μmol/L) had more than eight times the risk of kidney failure over five years when compared to those with normal uric acid levels. (See figure 2).[78] Also, two additional studies found that 79-99% of gout patients had kidney damage at the time of death.[84,85] Exactly what is happening to cause this kidney disease is not well understood, and there is some disagreement in the scientific literature about the strength of this association.[2]

In Chapter 2, kidney stones were mentioned as a risk of taking uricosuric drugs. However, the risk of urate kidney stones is also elevated in anyone with gout, particularly people who over-produce uric acid. Reports on the prevalence of kidney stones in people with gout varies considerably, but ranges from 6% to 40%.[6] Also, uric acid can help form kidney stones made of other substances.[9] Drinking 2-3 liters of water a day and regularly testing your urine pH can help prevent this. (See "Managing Hyperuricemia" in Chapter Two.)

Obesity: There is a strong link between hyperuricemia and body weight, due to the fact that obesity has been shown to weaken the kidneys' ability to remove uric acid, as well as increase production of uric acid. A few studies have suggested that hyperuricemia may actually cause obesity, but this has yet to be proven con-clusively.[78]

Stroke: Hyperuricemia has also been shown to be strongly associated with a poor outcome in stroke victims. A uric acid level above 7mg/dL (388μmol/L) is itself an independent risk factor for stroke and stroke deaths. Uric acid levels also increased the risk of later blood vessel problems in the brain. The risk is also significantly higher in people who are diabetic.[78]

Hypothyroidism: Hypothyroidism is a reduction in thyroid gland functioning. One study claims that as many as 15-20% of gout patients also have hypothyroid-ism, a rate significantly higher than those without gout, and high enough to sug-gest that thyroid screening should be done whenever gout is diagnosed.[2]

Cortical Cataracts: Cortical cataracts form in the lens of the eye and gradually extend "spokes" from the outside of the lens to the center. One study found the incidence of cortical cataracts to be higher in people who have had gout for more than 10 years.[86]

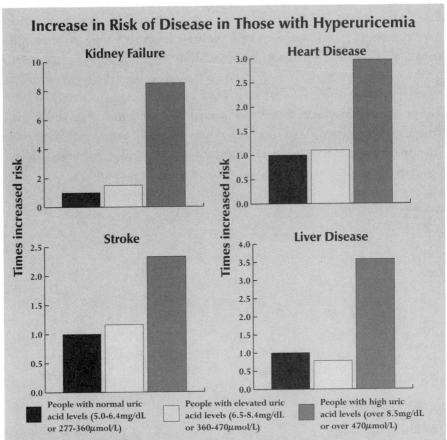

Figure 2: This chart shows the results of a large study of Japanese workers. In the study, higher uric acid levels were found to significantly increase the risk of heart disease, stroke and liver disease over five years. Overall, the largest risk was for kidney failure.[83]

Clearly, all of these are very serious conditions. It is not known whether hyperuricemia causes these conditions or is a symptom of them. Currently there is little scientific evidence that lowering uric acid levels will reduce the risk of any of these conditions;[6] more research needs to be done. But, the lack of evidence does not mean that reducing uric acid levels will not help, just that we do not know. The small amount of scientific research on the subject that does exist, however, suggests that positive health benefits do result from lowering uric acid levels.[7,79]

Hyperuricemia

The current practice is to not treat hyperuricemia that has not shown symptoms (i.e. gout).[6,19] However, there is growing doubt about this practice in the scientific literature,[13,70] and new research studies are underway to answer this question.[13]

Above all, the research shows that your hyperuricemia puts you at risk. You should be vigilant about these conditions and work to prevent them. Steps you can take to prevent these conditions, as well as lowering your uric acid levels and reducing gout attacks, will be the subject of the next chapter.

Chapter Five:

Diet and Lifestyle

"Be temperate in wine, in eating, girls, and sloth;
Or the Gout will seize you and plague you both"
- Benjamin Franklin

We have all heard it – "Eat right, lose weight and exercise." Most of us ignore this sage advice. For people suffering from gout, however, this could be a fatal error.[27] The previous chapter outlined the many life-threatening conditions that are associated with gout and hyperuricemia. As a gout sufferer, your chances of developing at least one of these conditions is exceptionally high. The good news is that for many people, this risk can be greatly reduced by following a careful diet, losing weight and engaging in regular exercise.[88]

Simple adjustments to your diet and lifestyle can significantly lower uric acid levels, reduce the need for medication and reduce the frequency of gout attacks. Even if you are not on uric acid-lowering medication, the advice in this chapter will help you lower your uric acid levels and improve your overall health.[7]

Weight and Exercise

The impact of weight control and exercise on uric acid levels and overall health cannot be overemphasized. Extra pounds cause both increased production of uric acid and reduced excretion.[70] It has been demonstrated that losing weight and lowering your body mass index (See Figure 1) can significantly reduce uric acid levels, lower blood pressure, and lower your risk of cardiovascular problems and stroke.

Losing weight and exercising regularly are also the best ways to fight Metabolic syndrome and many of the other conditions associated with hyperuricemia mentioned in the last chapter.[9,66,70,89,90,91] *If you are overweight, the single best thing you can do for your health (including your gout) is to exercise regularly, lose weight and keep it off.*[26,75,129,130]

The Centers for Disease Control and Prevention (CDC) recommends moderate exercise for at least 30 minutes a day, *five days a week* or vigorous exercise three days a week. Ask your doctor what the best type and level of exercise is for your current health condition, and do it! If it has been awhile, start slowly and work your way up as your endurance builds. It helps to consult a professional, such as a personal trainer, to establish your workout routine. Just be careful not to overdo it, since intense physical activity or joint trauma may aggravate gout. For most gout patients, moderate exercise is best.[26]

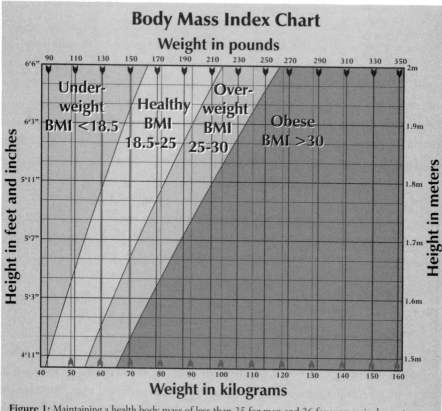

Figure 1: Maintaining a health body mass of less than 25 for men and 26 for women is shown to result in lower uric acid levels, reduced gout attacks and is a key predictor of how long you will live.[14]

One small study demonstrated the power of weight loss on gout. The participants had an average body mass index of 30.5 and were put on a balanced, reduced-calorie diet. They lost an average of 17 pounds each over the course of 16 weeks. As a result, their gout attacks decreased from an average of two per month to only .6 per month, while their serum uric acid levels decreased from

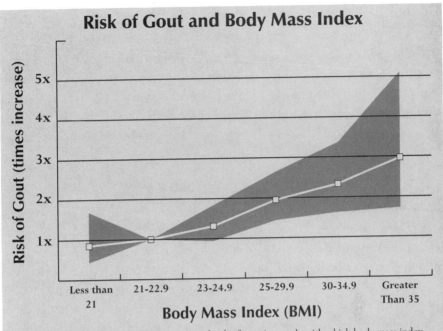

Figure 2: The chart below shows the increased risk of gout in people with a high body mass index when compared to a healthy BMI.[66] The line shows the mean value, and the gray area shows the possible range based on the available data.

an average of 10.26mg/dL (570μmol/L) to 8.45mg/dL (470μmol/L). More than half actually achieved normal uric acid levels without using any uric acid lowering medications. These patients also saw substantial improvements in other areas of their health, including significant reductions in their total cholesterol and triglycerides.[92]

There is nothing new about these findings. This is the same thing you hear from public health experts all the time. But in the case of the gout sufferer, losing weight and exercising becomes even more important. Your hyperuricemia predisposes you to many other health problems, not just gout. Preventing gout and lowering uric acid levels is one more (big) reason why you should make these changes in your lifestyle and make them permanent

For extremely obese people who have tried and failed to lose weight through diet and exercise, the anti-obesity drugs sibutramine (Trade names: Meridia® and Reductil®) and orlistat (Trade names: Xenical® and Alli®) have all been shown to result in lower uric acid levels, as has bariatric (weight loss) surgery.[78]

Alcohol

Alcohol is one of the most significant lifestyle factors that affects gout. Alcohol causes both an increase in the production of uric acid and a decrease in excretion.[93,94,95] It is also a diuretic (which causes the body to lose water), further increasing the concentration of uric acid in the body. This triple threat is why conventional medical wisdom has long held that people with gout should not drink *any* alcohol.[90]

In recent years, however, new research has shown that there is a bit more nuance to this wisdom than previously thought. Different types of alcoholic beverages impact gout to different degrees. New research has confirmed that consuming beer is the worst dietary choice you can make for hyperuricemia and gout. Drinking just one beer per day on average nearly *doubles* your risk of gout compared to those who do not drink. Averaging two beers per day will boost the risk up to two-and-a-half times. *People with gout should <u>not</u> drink beer.* Light or non-alcoholic beers carry the same risks for gout as regular beer. This means that there is something in beer other than the alcohol that makes it so bad for people with gout.[93,94]

Spirits such as vodka, gin and whisky are also bad for gout, but to a lesser degree than beer – the risk is a little more than half that of beer. A daily glass of red wine, meanwhile, has been shown to slightly reduce the risk of gout, with the risk being about even with those that do not drink, when drinking two glasses a day.[95]

Therefore, if you are going to consume any alcoholic beverages, stick to red wine, and limit yourself to one or two glasses per day. Some experts now recommend that people with gout consume one glass of red wine per day. One glass may not only slightly reduce your risk of gout, but it has also been strongly associated with a 25 to 40% reduction in the risk of coronary heart disease.[96] Therefore, if your doctor approves, adding a daily glass of red wine is a great way to relax at the end of the day, and as a bonus it may actually *improve* your health.

The key here is *moderation*. Gout sufferers are notoriously heavy drinkers; studies have shown that about half drink excessively.[9] *Never drink more than one or two drinks per day, and stick to red wine only.* Drinking more than this will cause your risk of an acute attack to go up rapidly. This effect is intensified if your BMI is over 25.[95]

Binge drinking and alcohol abuse has been shown to be worst of all. In addition to the three uric acid-raising effects of alcohol previously explained, many people who abuse alcohol fail to eat for lengthy periods of time and often forget to take their uric acid-lowering medications. Both of these actions exacerbate the effects of alcohol in increasing uric acid levels, making gout attacks much more likely.[9] Even worse, heavy alcohol consumption can reduce the effectiveness of allopurinol.[97]

Diet

Purines are the raw materials that the body metabolizes to create uric acid.[4] For many decades, conventional wisdom has held that in order to reduce uric acid levels you must reduce your intake of foods containing purines. This definitely is an effective way to reduce uric acid levels. However, new research has taken a closer look at the interplay between diet, Metabolic syndrome and hyperuricemia. In this research, subjects were given a diet tailored to preventing Metabolic syndrome, not avoiding purines. It was discovered that this diet was just as effective as a low purine diet at reducing uric acid levels, plus was considered more palatable. *In both cases, however, the effect on uric acid levels was fairly small.* Both diets reduced uric acid levels only about 1-2mg/dL (56-111μmol/l) of serum uric acid.[9,98,99]

So, which diet should you follow? That is a good question; unfortunately, no research yet exists that definitively proves which diet is better for gout management.[94] In many cases, hyperuricemia appears to be the result of a genetic predisposition, combined with poor diet and lifestyle habits that were learned early in life and never changed.

Over the years these poor habits allowed uric acid levels to increase and caused hyperuricemia to develop. Therefore, changing these habits may help alleviate this condition and remove some of the fuel for gout attacks, as well as improve a person's overall health.[6]

As for which diet to follow, this should be discussed with your doctor. If you are overweight or have other risk factors for Metabolic syndrome, then a diet tailored to losing weight and avoiding this syndrome would make sense for you.[6,70,94] This is especially true since low-purine diets usually are high in carbohydrates and saturated fats, which can increase your risk of diabetes and Metabolic syndrome.[92,100,101]

If you aren't overweight and are otherwise healthy, then a diet that avoids foods with a high purine content, along with reduced alcohol consumption and regular exercise, would probably be most beneficial.[6] The two diets are outlined below; however, you should always consult your doctor or a nutritionist to design a diet that is best for your particular situation.

Low Purine Diet

Information abounds on the Internet about low-purine diets. Scientists know the purine content of many foods, but no one really knows how different methods of preparation affect purine levels. This makes it difficult to know the exact quantity of purines you are ingesting.[90] Additionally, there are several different types of purines, each with different effects on uric acid levels.[102,103] For example, new research shows that moderate consumption of vegetables, even those high in purines, does not affect uric acid levels.[13] More research is needed to determine exactly which purines truly affect uric acid levels and what foods contain them. Meanwhile, it's recommended that you avoid the worst offenders and control your hyperuricemia with medication if needed. Strict low-purine diets should only be followed when medical conditions prevent you from using uric acid-lowering medications.[70]

Below is a list of foods that are high in purines, listed in order from highest to lowest. Appendix A contains a more complete list of food purine levels. No vegetables are listed below, as they do not affect uric acid levels and have additional health benefits:

Foods to avoid (highest purine content listed first):[26]
Foods made with baker's or brewer's yeast
Seafood: Sprat (smoked), sardines, canned herring, trout, mackerel, salmon, ocean perch (redfish) and shrimp
Organ Meats: Neck, spleen, lung, heart, liver, kidney, all other organ meats
Meats: Smoked meats[103]

Foods to eat sparingly:
Seafood: All other types not listed above including shellfish other than shrimp.
Meats: Chicken, veal, turkey, pork and all other meats

Foods with elevated levels of purines:
Nuts and seeds: (except poppy seeds and sunflower seeds). However, oils made from nuts have been shown to lower uric acid levels.
Fruits, except raisins
Grains, except barley and oats
Cheeses: All types

Diet to Prevent Metabolic Syndrome

If you have some or all of the symptoms of Metabolic syndrome or are at risk, you might consider switching to a diet designed to help prevent both this syndrome and insulin resistance. Your primary goal should be to reach your ideal weight by eating fewer calories along with the right kinds of foods.

Below are the main points of this diet, but again, you should consult a nutritionist to help you plan a diet tailored to your specific needs and tastes:[104]

- Reduce the number of calories you eat to lose weight as needed.
- Carbohydrates in foods are ranked on a scale called the *glycemic index,* based on their effect on blood glucose levels. Eat foods with a low glycemic index.
  - Examples of foods with a low glycemic index are: most fruits and vegetables (except potatoes, watermelon and sweet corn), whole grains, pasta, beans, lentils.
- Eat at least 20 grams of dietary fiber, especially soluble fiber, each day
- Eat six small meals instead of three large ones. This will reduce the amount of insulin released with each meal and lessen your chance of developing insulin resistance.
- Minimize the intake of food and beverages with high-fructose corn syrup and added sugars.
- Avoid foods rich in magnesium.
- Eat foods rich in vitamin C, beta-carotene, folate and vitamin B_{12}.
- Focus on eating more nuts and olive oil, which are good sources of heart-healthy fat. Just be sure to keep control of your calorie intake.
- Limit the amount of saturated fat, trans fat, cholesterol and sodium in your diet.
- Normally this diet recommends regular seafood consumption. Since seafood consumption can cause elevated uric acid levels, however, some experts have recommend replacing seafood consumption with plant-derived Omega-3 supplements or supplements of DHA (docahexaenoic acid) and EPA (eicosapentaenoic acid.)[45]
- Switch to fat-free and low-fat dairy products.
- Increase your physical activity.
- Avoid the use of and exposure to tobacco products.

Fad and Crash Diets

Eating plans such as the Atkin's diet™ remain popular, but have been found to increase uric acid levels, and thus the incidence of gout.[26,94] Also, "crash diets" or sudden, drastic reductions in calorie consumption have been shown to increase uric acid levels and trigger attacks.[88,105]

Unfortunately, there are no shortcuts to sustained weight loss. Managing weight by eating a balanced diet, gradually reducing your calorie intake and engaging in regular exercise is the best and most sustainable way to lose weight and keep it off.

Vitamin C

Vitamin C's impact on uric acid levels is strong. Research has demonstrated that taking 500 mg of vitamin C per day reduces uric acid levels by an average of 1.5mg/dL (83μmol/L) over two months.[106] Whether the effect is permanent is not known, but since vitamin C aids the kidneys in excreting uric acid (much as uricosuric drugs), it likely is.[13,107] Taking a multivitamin that contains 500 mg of vitamin C is a simple way to stay healthy and reduce uric acid levels.

However, vitamin C is a water-soluble acid, which may make your urine more acidic. Acidic urine increases the likelihood of urate kidney stones, particularly if you take uricosuric drugs such as probenecid.[108] If you decide to take vitamin C, drink plenty of water and check your urine pH regularly, as described in Chapter Two, to ensure against the formation of kidney stones.

Another study involving mega-doses of vitamin C (up to 8,000 mg/day) resulted in an even greater uric acid-lowering effect, up to 3.1mg/dL (172μmol/L). However, this study lasted only seven days and had only 14 subjects.[108] Such high levels of vitamin C might be dangerous if taken long term, and the rapid fluctuation in uric acid levels could actually spur gout attacks. Plus, the high level of uric acid excretion and acidification of urine can promote kidney stones. High doses of vitamin C can also interact with allopurinol and are thus not recommended.

Proteins, Dairy and Fats

For a long time gout suffers were told to avoid high-protein foods, because it was thought that these foods also contained high levels of purines. Research has demonstrated that this is not true.[102] In fact, a high-protein diet may actually reduce uric acid levels.[90,94,103,109]

The type of proteins consumed does make a difference. Meats are high in protein but increase uric acid levels. Fish, processed meats and beef are the worst offenders, followed by pork.[102] On the other hand, proteins from eggs, vegetables and soy – even those high in purines – can decrease uric acid levels. Some experts have suggested replacing all dietary fish with plant-derived Omega-3 supplements.[45]

Low-fat dairy products, particularly skimmed milk and low-fat yogurt, have been proven to lower uric acid levels significantly.[26,70,110] It is believed that this is the result of higher calcium intake, which has also been shown to reduce uric acid levels. However, testing on high-fat dairy products shows no effect on uric acid levels.[94]

One study revealed that people with the highest intake of low-fat dairy products had a 50% reduction in their risk of gout, compared to a group with a very low intake of dairy products.[70] Also, another study demonstrated that a diet free of all dairy products was associated with significantly higher uric acid levels.[102] If you cannot tolerate dairy products, some experts have suggested using calcium supplements as a substitute.[98,103]

Although research is not yet available directly testing the effects of different types of fat on uric acid levels, in general you should avoid foods that contain saturated fats and trans fats such as: dairy or meat fats, chocolate, coconuts, coconut milk, coconut oil, most margarines, vegetable shortening, partially hydrogenated vegetable oil, most fast foods, most deep-fried foods and most commercial baked goods. Saturated fats are associated with higher cholesterol, coronary heart disease, cancer, diabetes and obesity, as well as other health problems. Replace these with mono- or poly-unsaturated fats such as almonds, peanuts, most other nuts, olives, olive oil, canola oil, corn oil, safflower oil, cottonseed oil, soybeans and avocados.

Lastly, avoid consumption of foods that are diuretics and cause the body to lose water, such as: cranberry juice, asparagus, celery, eggplant, lemon, garlic, cucumbers and licorice. Consumption of these foods, as with all diuretics, can increase uric acid levels.[111]

Other Lifestyle Factors that Affect Gout

Temperature

Temperature extremes can have an important effect on uric acid crystallization in the body. Blood serum is considered "saturated" with uric acid when it reaches a level of 6.8mg/dL (378μmol/L) at normal body temperature (98.6°F or 37°C). Crystals are much less likely to form if your uric acid level is below this level at normal body temperature. However, if your temperature drops, this "saturation point" also drops; at 95°F (35°C), the saturation point drops to 6mg/dL (334μmol/L) and at 86°F (30°C) it drops even further, to only 4.5mg/dL (250μmol/L).[10]

This is why many gout attacks strike in the feet and hands, since temperatures are usually lower in the body's extremities. This is also why gout attacks typically come on in the middle of the night, since sleep lowers body temperature even more.[7,112] Furthermore, since the saturation point for uric acid is 6.8mg/dL (378μmol/L), this is why doctors target less than 6mg/dL (334μmol/L) for uric acid-lowering treatment. The lower the uric acid level, the larger the margin for fluctuations in uric acid levels and temperature, without the risk of triggering an attack.

This is a useful fact, particularly for people who live in cold climates or work outdoors. It's important to keep your hands and feet warm and dry at all times. In addition, it has been shown that long periods of cold are worse for gout than rapid fluctuations in temperature.[10] For example, you are more likely to get a gout attack when the weather has been fairly cold for several days, versus a shorter, very cold, period.

Lastly, hot, humid weather and exposure to hot environments have also been shown to trigger gout attacks. In hot and humid weather the body becomes dehydrated, causing an increase in uric acid concentration in the body. To prevent this, drink lots of water to stay well hydrated.[113,114]

Airline Travel and Other Low Pressure Environments

My work requires me to travel frequently. After several business trips I noticed when I arrived home, my gout would frequently act up. This was likely due to the reduced air pressure on airplanes: aircraft cabins are typically pressurized to the equivalent of about 7,000-8,000 feet. It has been suggested in the scientific literature that regular exposure to low pressures/high altitudes can trigger gout attacks, although I could not find any studies addressing this problem directly.[6]

Fructose

Fructose is a simple sugar found in many foods. It occurs naturally in items such as honey, fruit, berries and melons, and artificially in items such as white sugar and high-fructose corn syrup, one of the main ingredients in soft drinks and other sweets. Fructose has been shown to elevate uric acid levels and also to promote Metabolic syndrome. Gout sufferers should avoid foods high in fructose, particularly juices and soft drinks. Avoiding fructose-rich foods is also recommended to prevent insulin resistance and Metabolic syndrome.[13,90,117]

Coffee and Tea

Coffee and tea contain caffeine, which is classified as a purine. Researchers have attempted to determine if coffee and tea consumption resulted in increased uric acid levels. The research found that not only did coffee *not* increase uric acid levels but actually caused a *decrease* when four or more cups were consumed per day. It didn't matter if the coffee was caffeinated or decaffeinated; therefore it would seem that there is something else in coffee that affects uric acid levels. While this effect was unexpected, it was relatively small, decreasing uric acid levels by about .5mg/dL or 28μmol/L. Therefore, individuals probably should not start drinking coffee in an effort to manage gout. Tea on the other hand, was found not to have any effect on uric acid levels despite the fact that it is a diuretic, regardless of how much was consumed.[118]

Aspirin

Low-dose aspirin therapy (81mg/day) for heart problems has been shown to increase uric acid levels, but there is some doubt about the strength of this effect.[13] If you are on low-dose aspirin therapy, talk to your doctor to weigh the risks versus the benefits or to discuss alternatives. Though painful, gout attacks are usually preferred over heart attacks!

High-dose aspirin therapy, such as that used for headaches and other pain, has been shown to lower uric acid levels. But it is not recommended that you take high doses of aspirin on a regular basis, since stomach problems can occur.[4,6] High doses of aspirin can also interfere with probenecid, lowering its effectiveness and resulting in higher uric acid levels.

Lifestyle Changes: Sustain them to Manage Gout without Drugs

In some cases, uric acid levels return to normal in people who stop drinking alcohol, lose weight and exercise regularly, making this the only known way to manage gout without drugs.[6,32,70] Unfortunately, less than 20% of patients actually make these changes in a sustained way.[119] This means the other 80% are shortening and reducing the quality of their lives. Do you want to be one of them?

If you have hyperuricemia and gout, there is a good chance you are already well on your way to serious health problems. The good news is that much of the damage can be stopped or even reversed. It won't be easy, but you will be happier and healthier if you stick with it. And, remember, always check with your doctor before making changes to your diet and exercise routine.

Diet and

Vitamins:

- A multivitamin with 500 mg of vitamin C can lower uric acid levels.
- Take calcium supplements if you cannot eat dairy products.
- Replace seafood with plant-derived Omega-3 supplements such as flaxseed oil.
- **In all cases,** check with your doctor first!

Food Pyramid

Use Sparingly

Red meat raises uric acid levels.

Calcium and low-fat dairy lowers uric acid levels.

Seafood and high consumption of poultry increase uric acid levels.

Vegetables, even those high in purines, should be eaten in abundance.

Exercise builds strength and cardiovascular health.

Butter
Red Meat

Calcium
Supplements
Low-fat dairy

Fish
Poultry

Nuts

Vegetables
Eat in abundance.

Whole-grain foods
Eat at most meals.

Daily Exercise

Other factors:

Avoid high-purine foods.

If you are at risk for Metabolic syndrome, discuss your diet with your doctor.

Avoid diuretic foods.

Do not use fad or crash diets.

Lifestyle

For Gout

Figure 3: The Food Pyramid for gout. Below is a modified food pyramid with foods and other factors that have been shown to increase and decrease uric acid levels.[45]

Alcohol:

Beer - Do not drink!
Spirits - Avoid
Red Wine - in moderation does not affect uric acid levels or cause gout.
All cases: Drink in moderation (one drink per day of red wine maximum) and only with approval from your doctor!

Use Sparingly

Avoid foods with a high glycemic index.

High-fat dairy does not affect uric acid levels.

Pasta
Sweets
Potatoes
White Rice
White Bread

High-fat dairy

1 - 2 servings per day

Eggs
0 - 2 servings per day

Nuts and legumes are healthy sources of unsaturated fats and do not increase uric acid levels.

Legumes
1 - 3 servings per day

Fruit
2 - 3 servings per day

Plant oils may lower uric acid levels.

Plant oils (olive, canola, sunflower, peanut, other vegetable oils)
At most meals

If overweight, losing weight is the best way to control gout and stay healthy.

Weight Control

Other factors:

Keep your hands and feet warm at all times.
Drink lots of water (2 to 3 liters/day), especially in hot weather.
Avoid foods high in fructose (i.e. soft drinks).
Do not use low-dose aspirin therapy, unless instructed to do so by your doctor.

Chapter Six:

Alternative Medicine

"Love and gout are incurable"
- Mesner

Despite the successes of modern Western medicine, many people still look to alternatives in the hope of finding a more "natural" cure for what ails them. But the fact is, most natural cures do not work, and the ones that do usually are or already have been incorporated into mainstream medications.

Take colchicine for example. Colchicine comes from the bulb of the autumn crocus flower (scientific name: *Colchicum autumnale*).[9] This natural "herbal" substance has been used by doctors and medicine men/women for more than 2,000 years to treat gout, as have a host of other natural substances that did not work. Over time, colchicine survived because it actually did work, and it is still a staple of gout treatment today.

Despite colchicine's natural origins, it is highly toxic. Many people over the centuries have died as a result of the, "If a little bit is good for you, more must be better" line of thinking. *Even natural remedies can be very dangerous.*

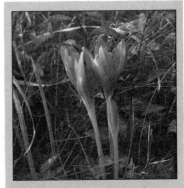

Photo: Colchicine is made from the bulb of this flower, the autumn crocus flower (formal name: Colchicum autumnale).
Photo by: Luc Viatour.

There are probably many other substances in nature that are beneficial to gout, but are unknown to modern medical science. It's more likely, though, that most of the currently known alternatives would have already been turned into medications by now if they actually worked. With the dangers that gout and hyperuricemia pose, it might not be worth taking the risk.

Anyone considering alternative medicines for gout should first talk to their doctor. Herbs, vitamins and everything else in nature is made of chemicals. These chemicals can react in unexpected ways with the ones in your other medications and in your body. Your doctor has spent years studying chemistry and the human body. He or she is the best person to decide which chemicals, even the naturally occurring ones, in alternative treatments are harmful, helpful or neutral, based on your medical history.[26]

Realizing that many gout patients are still interested in trying alternatives (and there is scientific evidence for some), I have listed some here. This list is by no means complete, and little effort has been made in the medical literature to cross check for interactions with prescription medications used to treat gout. Therefore, you should research these alternatives yourself and discuss them with your doctor, *before* using them.

If you know of an alternative medicine that you believe is effective, but is not listed here, please feel free to share it on this book's companion web site, http://www.beatinggout.com.

Alternative Treatments Backed by Scientific Evidence

Omega-3 fatty acids: Have been shown to reduce inflammation and can be used during a gout attack or as an alternative or supplement to colchicine for prophylaxis. This may reduce the frequency and intensity of gout attacks, but alone will not reduce uric acid levels.[13,88,98] Omega-3 fatty acids also have cardiovascular health benefits, namely lowering blood pressure and blood triglycerides. Typical dose: 1,600 mg per day for men and 1,100 mg per day for women.[120]

Vitamin E and Selenium: These are said to decrease inflammation and protect against joint damage caused by acute attacks. However, again they do not lower uric acid levels. Typical dose: Selenium, 55 micrograms per day (the daily recommended allowance), Vitamin E, 15 mg/day.[121]

Burdock Root: Burdock root was found to reduce the production of uric acid (along with the parts of many other trees) in one theoretical study which looked at the chemistry of the substances, but did not actually study them in humans.[122] However, I was not able to find any studies showing that Burdock root actually reduced uric acid levels in people. Burdock root is also a diuretic, which can increase uric acid concentrations, but it is not known which effect is stronger. Typical dose: one 475 mg tablet three times a day.[121] Teas made from burdock root, as well as other tree components, have also been suggested.

Reddish-blue berries such as Cherries, Blackberries, Hawthorn Berries and Elderberries and Cherry Juice: Flavonoids in these berries have been shown to lower uric acid levels and have an anti-inflammatory effect. However, the high fructose content may cancel some of the uric acid-lowering effect. About one cup of berries or 12 to 16 ounces of cherry juice per day is recommended.[13,123]

Ice: One study showed that applying ice to the affected joint during a gout attack can slow inflammation and reduce pain. This contradicts previous advice to keep the joints warm and dry. Warmth will prevent uric acid crystals from forming, but it can also speed inflammation once an attack starts. However, once an attack is underway, it's too late to prevent crystal formation, so the benefit of slowing the inflammation process may outweigh the risk of additional crystal formation.[19,26] Ice likely works best when the joint is also rested.

Alternative Treatments with Little or No Supporting Evidence

Folic Acid: More commonly known as vitamin B_9, folic acid is thought to inhibit the production of uric acid. It is recommended that you discuss this with your doctor and be monitored closely, as there is a high risk of adverse health effects. Typical dose: 400-800 micrograms per day. [121]

Garlic: Garlic has long been used in the treatment of gout and has many positive health benefits. However, there is little scientific data about its effectiveness against gout. *Also, garlic can promote bleeding, which makes it potentially very dangerous if you are also taking NSAIDs.* Typical dose: 600-900 mg of dehydrated garlic powder per day.[121]

Amino Acids: Amino acids, the building blocks of DNA, appear to increase the kidneys' ability to excrete uric acid. Recommended dosage is unknown.

Bromelain: Bromelain is an enzyme found in pineapples which has anti-inflammatory properties. It can be used during an attack or as a prophylactic to reduce the frequency and intensity of gout attacks, but it will not reduce uric acid levels. Typical dose: 200-400 mg, between meals, up to three times a day.

Celery Seed: In my research, I could not find any information on how celery seed impacts gout, but it appears frequently in alternative medicine references as a gout treatment, so it is included here. However, celery seed is a diuretic, which may increase uric acid levels. Celery seed is available in tablet form. Typical dose: 1,000 to 3,000 mg/day.

Devil's Claw: This herb is said to lower uric acid levels and relieve joint pain. Typical dose: up to 10 g of extract per day.

Ultrasound and chiropractic manipulative therapy: Ultrasound and chiropractic manipulative therapy have been suggested as a means of breaking up urate crystals. However, no studies confirm this, and I doubt these can have any lasting beneficial effect, as they may aggravate the inflammation of gout.

Homeopathic Therapies: Homeopathic therapies, in my opinion, do not work. This statement is backed up by numerous scientific studies. The most recent is a study appearing in *The Lancet*, one of the world's most respected medical journals.

Looking at 110 homeopathic trials, this study found that homeopathic treatments are no more effective then a placebo.[124] There have also been calls in the medical literature for doctors to come out and publicly rebuke these treatments, as their ineffectiveness has been definitively proven by the data.[125]

The idea behind homeopathic treatments is to take a substance that is "bad" for the targeted illness, and to dilute it in water many, many times. The resulting solution is than given as the remedy. As one book puts it, "Homeopathic remedies are frequently administered in minute, incomprehensibly small doses. For example, take a 2-liter bottle of soda, empty it into the Atlantic Ocean, stir, and take one teaspoonful. That dose – and doses far more dilute – can and do heal!"[126]

Using this process, it is highly unlikely that even one molecule of the medicinal substance would be in the remedy – meaning the "cure" is just plain water. For example, a "6C" dilution ("C" notation is used to describe the dilution factor in homeopathy) results in a remedy consisting of one part of the original substance in 1,000,000,000,000 (one trillion) parts of water. Remedies far more dilute are very common. The theory is that the water somehow "remembers" the presence of the offending substance, and this in turn triggers the body's natural immune system.

Another telling quote from this same book states, "How homeopathic remedies work, and if they are prepared in such tiny, tiny amounts, how could they possibly do anything in the body?" … Today, much research is being conducted on the international level. To date, however, no results have been forthcoming. We really don't know how homeopathic remedies work." The authors of *The Lancet* study mentioned above reviewed 110 such studies and found NO evidence that homeopathic remedies work.[126]

Therefore I suggest if you see the word "homeopathic" on a product, stay away from it, as you're probably paying good money for nothing more than plain water in a fancy package.

Appendix

Appendix A: Purine Content of Food

As mentioned before, it's difficult to know exact quantity of purines contained in any given food because different styles of preparation can change their concentration. Further, there are different types of purines, and science has not yet worked out exactly how each type affects uric acid levels. Despite the limitations of this data, it is the best that is available.

The quantities given below are in milligrams of uric acid per 100 grams of food.

Beverages:

Beer, light[1]	14
Beer, no alcohol[1]	3
Beer, pilsner[1]	13

Cheese & Yogurt:

Cheese, brie[1]	7
Cheese, camembert[1]	4
Cheese, cheddar[1]	7
Cheese, cottage[2]	8
Cheese, limburger[1]	32
Cheese, processed[2]	2
Yogurt, plain[2]	7

Fish & Shellfish:

Anchovies, canned[3]	321
Anchovies, raw[3]	411
Carp[1]	160
Caviar[1]	144
Caviar substitute[1]	18
Clams, canned[3]	62
Clams, raw[3]	136
Coalfish (saithe)[1]	60
Cod[1]	109
Crayfish[1]	60
Eel[1]	139
Eel, smoked[1]	78

Fish, canned[2]	206
Haddock, boiled[4]	95
Haddock, boiled--juice only[4]	23
Haddock, broiled[4]	119
Haddock, broiled[5]	193
Haddock, raw[4]	102
Halibut, cod & haddock[2]	125
Herring, canned[3]	378
Herring, roe[1]	190
Lobster[1]	118
Mackerel, canned[3]	246
Mackerel, raw[3]	194
Mussels[1]	112
Ocean perch (redfish)[1]	241
Oysters, canned[3]	107
Pike[1]	140
Pike perch[1]	110
Plaice[1]	93
Salmon, canned[3]	88
Salmon, raw[3]	250
Sardines, canned[3]	399
Sardines, raw[3]	345
Scallops[1]	136
Shellfish, unspecified[2]	72
Shrimp, canned[3]	234
Sole[1]	131

Sprat, smoked[1]	840
Squid, raw[3]	135
Trout[1]	297
Tuna, canned[3]	142
Whitefish, frozen[2]	129
Whitefish, raw[2]	116

Fruit:

Apples, raw[1]	14
Apricots, dried[1]	73
Avocados, raw[1]	19
Bananas, raw[1]	57
Bilberries, raw[1]	22
Cantaloupe, raw[1]	33
Cherries, morello, raw[1]	17
Cherries, sweet, raw[1]	17
Currants, red, raw[1]	17
Dates, dried[1]	35
Elderberries, raw[1]	33
Figs, dried[1]	64
Gooseberries, raw[1]	16
Grapes, raw[1]	27
Kiwifruit, raw[1]	19
Oranges, raw[1]	19
Peaches, raw[1]	21
Pears, raw[1]	12
Pineapples, raw[1]	19
Plums, dried[1]	64
Plums, raw[1]	24
Raisins[1]	107
Raspberries, raw[1]	18
Quince, raw[1]	30
Strawberries, raw[1]	21

Grains:

Barley, whole grain w/o husk[1]	94
Millet, shucked grain[1]	62
Oats, whole grain w/o husk[1]	94

Rice, white, cooked[2]	6
Rye, whole grain[1]	51
Wheat flour[2]	12
Wheat, whole grain[1]	51

Grain Products:

Bread, crusty[2]	16
Bread, white[2]	12
Corn cereal[2]	1
Crispbread[1]	60
Pasta, w/egg, dry[1]	40
Rolls[1]	21
Waffles/pancakes[2]	4

Meats:

Beef brisket[1]	90
Beef chunk[1]	120
Beef fillet[1]	110
Beef forerib[1]	120
Beef, ground[2]	90
Beef, roast[2]	125
Beef, roast & stew[2]	109
Beef rump[1]	120
Beef roast (sirloin)[1]	110
Beef shoulder[1]	110
Beef sirloin[4]	125
Beef steak, boiled[4]	108
Beef steak, boiled--juice only[4]	59
Beef steak, broiled[4]	121
Beef steak, raw[4]	106
Lamb roast & chops[2]	128
Pork, cured[2]	86
Pork chop[1]	145
Pork chunk[1]	140
Pork fillet[1]	150
Pork hip bone (hind leg)[1]	120
Pork leg (hind leg)[1]	160
Pork roast, chops[2]	120

Pork sausage[1]	101
Pork shoulder[1]	150
Veal chop, cutlet[1]	140
Veal cutlet[2]	143
Veal knuckle[1]	150
Veal leg[1]	150
Veal neck[1]	150
Veal sausage[1]	91
Veal shoulder[1]	140

Meats – Game:

Hare[1]	105
Horse[1]	200
Rabbit[1]	132
Venison, back[1]	105
Venison, leg[1]	138

Meats – Organ/Other:

Belly, pork[1]	100
Belly, pork, raw, smoked/dried[1]	127
Brains, beef[3]	162
Brains, calf[1]	92
Brains, ox[1]	75
Brains, pork[1]	83
Heart, beef[3]	171
Heart, lamb[3]	171
Heart, ox[1]	256
Heart, pork[1]	530
Heart, sheep[1]	241
Kidney, beef[3]	213
Kidney, calf[1]	218
Kidney, ox[1]	269
Kidney, pork[1]	334
Liver, beef, boiled[4]	237
Liver, beef, boiled--juice only[4]	49
Liver, beef, broiled[4]	236
Liver, beef, raw[4]	202
Liver, calf[1]	460
Liver, lamb[3]	147

Liver, ox[1]	554
Liver, pork[3]	289
Lung, calf[1]	147
Lung, ox[1]	399
Lung, pork[1]	434
Spleen, calf[1]	343
Spleen, ox[1]	444
Spleen, pork[1]	516
Spleen, sheep[1]	773
Neck, calf[1]	1260
Tongue, ox[1]	160
Tongue, pork[1]	136

Meats – Luncheon:

Bierschinken sausage[1]	85
Black pudding (blutwurst)[1]	55
Cold cuts[2]	70
Corned beef[1]	57
Fleischwurst (sausage)[1]	78
Frankfurters[1]	89
Jagdwurst (sausage)[1]	112
Liverwurst (liver sausage)[1]	165
Luncheon meat[2]	58
Ham, cooked[1]	131
Mettwurst (sausage)[1]	74
Mortadella[1]	96
Munich weibwurst (sausage)[1]	73
Salami[1]	104
Vienna sausage[1]	78

Nuts & Seeds:

Almonds[1]	37
Brazil nuts[1]	23
Hazelnuts[1]	37
Peanuts[1]	79
Walnuts[1]	25
Poppy seeds, dry[1]	170
Sesame seeds, dry[1]	62
Sunflower seeds, dry[1]	143

Poultry:

Chicken, broiler, breast[7]	131
Chicken, broiler, breast, raw[8]	168
Chicken, broiler, breast, roasted[8]	179
Chicken, broiler, drumstick[7]	132
Chicken, broiler, gizzard[7]	131
Chicken, broiler, liver[7]	236
Chicken, broiler, neck & back[7]	94
Chicken, broiler, neck[7]	123
Chicken, broiler, skin[7]	105
Chicken, broiler, thigh[7]	127
Chicken, broiler, thigh, raw[7]	152
Chicken, broiler, thigh, roasted[7]	149
Chicken heart[3]	223
Chicken liver[3]	243
Chicken, roaster[1]	115
Chicken, stewer, breast, raw[6]	178
Chicken, stewer, breast, stewed[6]	184
Chicken, stewer, skin, raw[6]	59
Chicken, stewer, skin, stewed[6]	94
Chicken, stewer, thigh, raw[6]	144
Chicken, stewer, thigh, stewed[6]	146
Duck[1]	138
Goose[1]	165
Turkey w/skin[1]	150

Vegetables:

Artichokes, raw[1]	78
Asparagus, raw[1]	23
Bamboo shoots, raw[1]	29
Beets, raw[1]	19
Broccoli, raw[1]	81
Brussels sprouts, raw[1]	69
Cabbage, Chinese, raw[1]	21
Cabbage, red, raw[1]	32
Cabbage, savory, raw[1]	37
Cabbage, white, raw[1]	22
Carrots, raw[1]	17
Cauliflower, raw[1]	51
Celeriac (celery root), raw[1]	30
Chicory, raw[1]	12
Chives, raw[1]	67
Corn, raw[1]	52
Cress, raw[1]	28
Cucumbers, raw[1]	7
Eggplant, raw[1]	21
Endive, raw[1]	17
Fennel leaves, raw[1]	14
Kale, raw[1]	48
Kohlrabi, raw[1]	25
Lamb's lettuce, raw[1]	38
Leeks, raw[1]	74
Lettuce, raw[1]	13
Mushrooms, boletus, dried[1]	488
Mushrooms, boletus, raw[1]	92
Mushrooms, chanterelle, canned[1]	6
Mushrooms, chanterelle, raw[1]	17
Mushrooms, canned[2]	25
Mushrooms, morel, raw[1]	30
Mushrooms, oyster, raw[1]	50
Onions, raw[1]	13
Parsley, raw[1]	57
Peppers, green, raw[1]	55
Potatoes, raw[1]	16
Potatoes, cooked w/skin[1]	18
Pumpkin, raw[1]	44
Radishes, small, raw[1]	13
Rhubarb, raw[1]	12
Salsify, black, raw (oyster plant)[1]	71
Sauerkraut, raw[1]	16
Soybean sprouts, raw[1]	80
Spinach, raw[1]	57
Tomatoes, raw[1]	11
Zucchini, raw[1]	24

Vegetables – Legumes:

Chickpeas, dry[3]	56
Cowpeas, dry[3]	230
Cranberry beans, dry[3]	75
French beans[1]	37
French beans, dry[1]	45
Great Northern beans, dry[3]	213
Green peas[1]	84
Lentils, dry[3]	222
Lima beans, baby, dry[3]	114
Lima beans, large, dry[3]	149
Linseed[1]	105
Mungo beans, dry[1]	222
Peas, split, dry[3]	195
Pinto beans, dry[3]	171
Red beans, dry[3]	162
Soybeans, boiled[5]	185
Tofu[1]	68
White beans, small, dry[3]	202

Miscellaneous:

Cocoa powder[1]	71
Olives, green, marinated[1]	29
Soup w/meat[2]	12
Yeast, baker's, compressed[1]	680
Yeast, brewer's, dried[1]	1810

Sources:

[1] Souci SW, Fachmann HK, *et al.* Food Composition and Nutritional Tables. Stuttgart: Medpharm GmbH Scientific Publishers. 2000.

[2] Brule D, *et al.* Purine content of selected canadian food products. Journal of Food Composition Analysis. 1988;1:130-138.

[3] Clifford AJ, *et al.* Levels of purines in foods and their metabolic effects in rats. Journal of Nutrition. 1976;106:435-442.

[4] Brule D, *et al.* Effects of methods of cooking on free and total purine bases in meat and fish. Journal of Inst Can Sci Technology Aliment 1989;22:248-251.

[5] Brule D, *et al.* Changes in serum uric acid levels in normal human subjects fed purine-rich foods containing different amounts of adenine and hypoxanthine. Journal of American Coll Nutrition. 1992;11:353-358.

[6] Young LL. Effect of stewing on purine content of broiler tissue. Journal of Food Science. 1983;48:315-316.

[7] Young LL. Evaluation of four purine compounds in poultry products. Journal of Food Science. 1980;45:1064-1067.

[8] Young LL. Purine content of raw and roasted chicken broiler meat. Journal of Food Science. 1982;47:1374-1375.

Appendix B: Additional Information on Medications

Important note: This appendix contains additional information on several of the medications mentioned in this book, as well as other medications that are in late-stage clinical research trials or are available for special cases. This information is intended to supplement, not substitute for, the expertise and judgment of your physician, pharmacist or other health care professional. *Always* read drug information provided by your pharmacist or health care provider. This information is *not* intended to imply that the use of these medications is safe, appropriate or effective for you. *Consult your doctor before taking any of these medications.*

General Information on Non-Steroidal Anti-Inflammatory Medications (NSAIDs):[36]

Below you will find general information put out by the FDA that applies to all NSAIDs. Please read this information carefully, and discuss any concerns you have with your doctor prior to taking any NSAIDs.

• • •

NSAID medicines may increase the chance of a fatal heart attack or stroke. This chance increases with long-term use of NSAID medicines and is higher for people who have heart disease.

NSAID medicines should never be used directly before or after coronary artery bypass graft (CABG) heart surgery.

NSAID medicines can cause ulcers and bleeding in the stomach and intestines at any time during treatment. Ulcers and bleeding can happen without warning symptoms and may cause death.

The chance of a person developing an ulcer or bleeding increases with:
- Taking medicines called "corticosteroids" and "anti-coagulants"
- Longer use
- Smoking
- Drinking alcohol
- Older age
- Overall poor health

NSAID medicines should only be used:
- Exactly as prescribed
- At the lowest dose possible for your treatment
- For the shortest time needed

Do not take an NSAID medicine if you have had an asthma attack, hives or other allergic reaction to aspirin or any other NSAID medicine right before or after heart bypass surgery.

Tell your health care provider about all of your medical conditions, and all of the medicines you take, even over-the-counter varieties and vitamin/herbal supplements. NSAIDs and some other medicines can interact with each other and cause serious side effects. Keep a current written list of your medicines to show to your health care provider and pharmacist.

Pregnant women should not use NSAID medicines late in their pregnancy (the third trimester). If you are breast-feeding, talk to your doctor before taking any NSAID.

Serious side effects of NSAIDs include:
- Heart attack
- Stroke
- High blood pressure
- Heart failure from body swelling (fluid retention)
- Kidney problems including kidney failure
- Bleeding and ulcers in the stomach and intestine
- Low red blood cells (anemia)
- Life-threatening skin reactions
- Life-threatening allergic reactions
- Liver problems including liver failure
- Asthma attacks in people who have asthma

Other side effects include:
- Stomach pain
- Constipation
- Diarrhea
- Gas
- Heartburn
- Nausea
- Vomiting
- Dizziness

Get emergency help right away if you have any of the following symptoms: shortness of breath or trouble breathing, chest pain, weakness in one part or side of your body, slurred speech or swelling of the face or throat.

Stop your NSAID medicine and call your health care provider right away if you have any of the following symptoms: nausea, more tired or weaker than usual, itching, your skin or eyes look yellow, stomach pain, flu-like symptoms, if you vomit blood, there is blood in your bowel movement or it is black and sticky like tar, have unusual weight gain, skin rash or blisters with fever or swelling of the arms and legs, hands and feet.

These are not all of the side effects that can occur with NSAID medicines. Talk to your healthcare provider or pharmacist for more information about these drugs.

Aspirin is an NSAID medicine but it does not increase your chance of a heart attack. Aspirin can cause bleeding in the brain, stomach and intestines. It can also cause ulcers in the stomach and intestines.

Some of these NSAID medicines are sold in lower doses without a prescription (over-the-counter). Talk to your health care provider before using over-the-counter NSAIDs for more than 10 days.

• • •

Information on Specific NSAIDs:[461]

Indomethacin _____

Use: NSAID used to treat acute gout. May also be used as a prophylactic to prevent gout attacks.

Trade names include: Apo-Indomethacin®, Indameth®, Indocid®, Indocin®, Indo-Lemmon®, Indomethagan®, Arthrexin®, Indocid®, Novo-Methacin®

Tell you doctor if any of these apply to you *before* taking this medication:
- If you are anemic
- If you have asthma, especially aspirin-sensitive asthma
- If you have bleeding problems or are taking medicines that make you bleed more easily, such as anticoagulants (also known as "blood thinners")
- If you smoke cigarettes
- If you have had coronary artery bypass graft (CABG) surgery within the past two weeks
- If you have a dental disease
- If you are depressed
- If you have diabetes
- If you drink more than three alcoholic beverages a day
- If you have heart or circulation problems such as angina, high blood pressure, heart failure, heart rhythm problems, history of heart attack, history of blood clots or fluid retention in the legs
- If you have kidney disease
- If you have liver disease
- If you have Parkinson's disease
- If you have seizures or convulsions
- If you have stomach or duodenal ulcers
- If you have a history of stroke
- If you have systemic lupus erythematosus
- If you have ulcerative colitis
- If you have ever had an unusual or allergic reaction to indomethacin, aspirin, other salicylates, other NSAIDs, foods, dyes or preservatives
- If you are pregnant or trying to get pregnant
- If you are breast-feeding

Indomethacin

Drugs and herbal products that can interact with indomethacin:

- Abciximab
- Alcohol
- Alendronate
- Aminoglycosides
- Aspirin and aspirin-containing medicines
- Cefamandole
- Cefoperazone
- Cidofovir
- Clopidogrel
- Cyclosporine
- Drospirenone; ethinylestradiol (Yasmin®)
- Digoxin
- Entecavir
- Eptifibatide
- Lithium
- Medicines for high blood pressure
- Medicines that affect platelets
- Medicines that treat or prevent blood clots, such as Warfarin and other "blood thinners"
- Methotrexate
- Other anti-inflammatory drugs, including other NSAIDs (such as ibuprofen and prednisone)
- Pemetrexed
- Penicillamine
- Phenytoin
- Plicamycin
- Ticlopidine
- Tirofiban
- Water pills (diuretics)
- Valproic acid
- Zidovudine
- Herbal products that contain feverfew, garlic, ginger, ginkgo biloba, anise, arnica, bogbean, chamomile, chondroitin, clove, dong quai, ginseng, arginine, gossypo, bearberry and bilberry

Indomethacin _____

Other Information:

- Probenecid can increase the potency of indomethacin. If you take probenecid, discuss the correct dose of indomethacin with your doctor.
- Do not take any new medications, including over-the-counter medications, while taking indomethacin without talking to a doctor first.
- Do not drink alcohol, take aspirin or aspirin-containing medications, or any other anti-inflammatory medications without first talking to your doctor.
- Use exactly as prescribed.
- Take medicines with food, milk or antacid to reduce the chance of gastrointestinal problems.
- Drink lots of fluids (2-3 liters/day) unless on a fluid-restricted diet.
- Use caution when driving or performing tasks where alertness is needed, until you know how this medication affects you.
- Eating small, frequent meals, chewing gum or sucking on lozenges may help if heartburn occurs.
- If taking medications long term, weigh yourself weekly, and report any unusual weight gain (more than 3-5 pounds or 1-2 kg per week) to your doctor.

Side Effects:

- Drowsiness
- Dizziness
- Nervousness
- Headache
- Decreased appetite
- Nausea
- Vomiting
- Heartburn
- Fluid Retention
- Green urine (This is normal when taking indomethacin.)

Indomethacin _____

Severe gastrointestinal bleeding, ulceration or perforation, or heart problems may occur at any time, with or without warning or pain. Contact your doctor immediately if you have any of these side effects:

- Persistent abdominal pain or cramping
- Rapid heartbeat or palpitations
- Unusual bruising or bleeding
- Difficulty breathing
- Unusual cough
- Chest pain
- Blood in your urine, stool, mouth or vomit
- Swollen extremities
- Skin rash, irritation or itching
- Acute fatigue
- Changes in vision, hearing or ringing in the ears
- Depression or anxiety
- Increased joint pain
- Fever

Naproxen _____

Use: NSAID used to treat acute gout. May also be used as a prophylactic to prevent gout attacks.

Trade names include: Aleve®, Naprosyn®, Anaprox®, Anaprox DS®, Apo-Naproxen®, Naxen®, Novo-Naprox®, Nu-Naprox®, Naprelan®

Tell your doctor if any of these apply to you *before* taking this medication:

- If you are anemic
- If you have asthma, especially aspirin-sensitive asthma
- If you have bleeding problems or are taking medicines that make you bleed easily, such as anticoagulants ("blood thinners")
- If you smoke cigarettes
- If you have had coronary artery bypass graft (CABG) surgery within the past two weeks
- If you have diabetes
- If you drink more than three alcoholic beverages a day
- If you have heart or circulation problems, such as angina, high blood pressure, heart failure, heart rhythm problems, a history of heart attack or a history of blood clots

93

Naproxen

- If you have kidney disease
- If you have liver disease
- If you have stomach or digestive system ulcers
- If you have a history of stroke
- If you have systemic lupus erythematosus
- If you have ulcerative colitis
- If you have ever had an unusual or allergic reaction to naproxen, aspirin, other salicylates, other NSAIDs, other medicines, foods, dyes or preservatives
- If you are pregnant or trying to get pregnant
- If you are breast-feeding

Drugs and herbal products that can interact with Naproxen:

- Alcohol
- Alendronate
- Aspirin and aspirin-containing medicines
- Cefamandole
- Cefotetan
- Cefoperazone
- Cidofovir
- Clopidogrel
- Corticosteroids
- Cyclosporine
- Entecavir
- Eptifibatide
- Lithium
- Medicines for high blood pressure
- Medicines that affect platelets
- Medicines that treat or prevent blood clots, such as Warfarin and other "blood thinners"
- Methotrexate
- Other anti-inflammatory drugs, such as ibuprofen or prednisone
- Pemetrexed
- Plicamycin
- Ticlopidine
- Tirofiban

Naproxen

- Valproic acid
- Water pills (diuretics)
- Herbal products that contain feverfew, garlic, ginger, ginkgo biloba, anise, arnica, bogbean, chamomile, chondroitin, clove, dong quai, fenugreek, ginseng, licorice, arginine, gossypo, bearberry and bilberry

Other Information:

- Do not take any new medications, including over-the-counter medications while taking this one without talking to a doctor first.
- Do not drink alcohol, take aspirin or aspirin-containing medications, or take any other anti-inflammatory medications without talking to your doctor first.
- Use exactly as prescribed.
- Take with food or milk to reduce the chance of gastrointestinal problems. (However, taking Naproxen on an empty stomach will speed absorption.)
- Drink lots of fluids (2-3 liters/day) unless on a fluid-restricted diet.
- Use caution when driving or performing tasks where alertness is needed until you know how this medication affects you.
- Eating small, frequent meals, chewing gum or sucking on lozenges may help if heartburn occurs.
- If taking Naproxen long term, weigh yourself weekly, and report any unusual weight gain (more than 3-5 pounds or 1-2 kg per week) to your doctor.
- This medication may increase your sensitivity to the sun. Use sunscreen if you will be spending time outdoors.

Side Effects:

- Drowsiness
- Dizziness
- Lightheadedness
- Nervousness
- Headache
- Decreased appetite
- Nausea
- Vomiting
- Heartburn
- Fluid retention

Naproxen

Severe gastrointestinal bleeding, ulceration or perforation, or heart problems may occur at any time, with or without warning or pain. Contact your doctor *immediately* if you have any of these side effects:

- Persistent abdominal pain or cramping
- Rapid heartbeat or palpitations
- Breathlessness
- Difficulty breathing
- Unusual cough
- Chest pain
- Unusual bruising or bleeding
- Blood in the urine, stool, mouth or vomit
- Swollen extremities
- Skin rash, irritation or itching
- Acute fatigue
- Changes in vision, hearing or ringing in the ears
- Increased joint pain
- Fever
- Flu-like symptoms
- Black, tarry stools

Sulindac

Use: NSAID used to treat acute gout.

Trade names include: Clinoril®, Aclin®, Apo-Sulin®, Novo-Sundac®

Tell your doctor if any of these apply to you *before* taking this medication:

- If you are anemic
- If you have asthma, especially aspirin-sensitive asthma
- If you have bleeding problems or are taking medicines that make you bleed more easily, such as anticoagulants (also known as "blood thinners")
- If you smoke cigarettes
- If you have had coronary artery bypass graft (CABG) surgery within the past two weeks
- If you have diabetes
- If you drink more than three alcoholic beverages a day

Sulindac

- If you have heart or circulation problems, such as angina, high blood pressure, heart failure, heart rhythm problems, a history of heart attack, a history of blood clots, or fluid retention in the legs
- If you have kidney disease
- If you have liver disease
- If you have stomach or digestive system ulcers
- If you have a history of stroke
- If you have systemic lupus erythematosus
- If you have ulcerative colitis
- If you have ever had an unusual or allergic reaction to indomethacin, aspirin, other salicylates, other NSAIDs, foods, dyes or preservatives
- If you are pregnant or trying to get pregnant
- If you are breast-feeding

Drugs and herbal products that can interact with sulindac:
- Alcohol
- Aspirin and aspirin-containing medicines
- Cidofovir
- Clopidogrel
- Corticosteroids
- Cyclosporine
- Entecavir
- Eptifibatide
- Lithium
- Medicines for high blood pressure
- Medicines that affect platelets
- Medicines that treat or prevent blood clots, such as Warfarin and other "blood thinners"
- Medications used to treat diabetes (Sulfonylureas)
- Methotrexate
- Other anti-inflammatory drugs (such as diflunisal, ibuprofen or prednisone)
- Pemetrexed
- Plicamycin
- Probenecid
- Some antibiotics (including some cephalosporins)
- Ticlopidine

Sulindac _____

- Tirofiban
- Valproic acid
- Water pills (diuretics)
- Herbal products that contain bogbean, chondroitin, arginine, gossypo, bearberry and bilberry

Other Information:

- Probenecid can increase the toxicity of sulindac. If you take probenecid, discuss this with your doctor.
- Do not take any new medications, including over-the-counter medications, while taking this one without talking to a doctor first.
- Do not drink alcohol, take aspirin or aspirin-containing medications or any other anti-inflammatory medications without talking to your doctor first.
- Use exactly as prescribed.
- Take with food or milk, to reduce the chance of gastrointestinal problems.
- Drink lots of fluids (2-3 liters/day) unless on a fluid-restricted diet.
- Use caution when driving or performing tasks where alertness is needed until you know how this medication affects you.
- Eating small, frequent meals, chewing gum or sucking on lozenges may help if heartburn occurs.
- If taking sulindac long term, weigh yourself weekly, and report any unusual weight gain (more than 3-5 pounds or 1-2 kg per week) to your doctor.
- This medication may increase your sensitivity to the sun. Use sunscreen if you will be spending time outdoors.
- Take this medication with a full glass of water.

Side Effects:

- Dizziness
- Nervousness
- Headache
- Nausea
- Vomiting
- Heartburn
- Constipation

Sulindac _____

Severe gastrointestinal bleeding, ulceration, perforation or heart problems may occur at any time, with or without warning or pain. Contact your doctor *immediately* if you have any of these side effects:

- Persistent abdominal pain or cramping
- Breathlessness
- Difficulty breathing
- Chest pain
- Unusual bruising or bleeding
- Blood in your urine, stool, mouth or vomit
- Swollen extremities
- Skin rash, irritation or itching
- Change in urination patterns
- Changes in vision, hearing or ringing in the ears
- Increased joint pain
- Fever

Information on Colchicine:

Use: Used to treat acute gout. May also be used as a prophylactic to prevent gout attacks. (Note: Colchicine is not a NSAID.)

Tell you doctor if any of these apply to you *before* taking this medication:

- If you have an alcohol abuse problem
- If you have any blood disorders
- If you have any dental disease
- If you are having any intramuscular injections
- If you have heart disease
- If you have kidney disease
- If you have liver disease
- If you have any stomach or intestinal disease
- If you have had any unusual or allergic reactions to colchicine, other medicines, foods, dyes or preservatives
- If you are pregnant or trying to get pregnant
- If you are breast-feeding

Colchicine _____

Drugs and herbal products that can interact with colchicine:
- Alcohol
- Anti-inflammatory drugs (NSAIDs, such as ibuprofen)
- Bone marrow depressants
- Clarithromycin
- Cyclosporine
- Erythromycin
- Vitamin B$_{12}$

Other Information:
- Use exactly as prescribed.
- Never exceed the recommended dose.
- Drink lots of fluids (2-3 liters/day) unless on a fluid-restricted diet.
- Do not drink alcohol or over-the-counter medications that contain alcohol
- Do not take aspirin or aspirin-containing medications without talking to your doctor first.
- You may experience temporary hair loss while on this medication.
- Bone marrow depression may occur while on this medication, increasing your risk of infection and/or anemia.
- Be sure to take any other medications your doctor has prescribed.
- This medication may suppress your ability to absorb vitamin B$_{12}$; therefore you may require vitamin B$_{12}$ supplementation by injection.
- Do not use colchicine to treat acute attacks if you are taking a daily dose (prophylaxis).

Side Effects:
- Nausea
- Vomiting
- Diarrhea
- Decreased appetite

Contact your doctor *immediately* if you have any of these side effects:
- Pain, redness or hard areas, especially on the legs
- Difficulty breathing[19]
- Rash
- Sore throat

Colchicine _____

- Fever
- Bleeding
- Weakness
- Numbness
- Tingling

Uric Acid Lowering Medications:

Allopurinol _____

Use: Works to treat gout by lowering serum uric acid levels. Allopurinol is a xanthine oxidase inhibitor drug, which prevents uric acid synthesis.

Trade names include: Lopurin®, Zyloprim®, Allorin®, Capurate®, Apo-Allopurinol®

Tell your doctor if any of these apply to you *before* **taking this medication:**
- If you have kidney disease
- If you have liver disease
- If you have ever had an unusual or allergic reaction to allopurinol, other medicines, foods, dyes or preservatives
- If you are pregnant or trying to get pregnant
- If you are breast-feeding

Drugs and herbal products that can interact with allopurinol:
- Ammonium chloride (found in some cold medicines)
- Vitamin C
- Potassium phosphate
- Sodium phosphate (a food preservative)
- Ampicillin
- Amoxicillin
- Medications used to treat diabetes
- Medications used to treat hypertension or congestive heart failure (ACE inhibitors and thiazides)

Allopurinol

- Medications to treat cancer (antineoplastics such as mercaptopurine and azathioprine)
- Theophylline

Other Information:
- Take only as prescribed. If you miss a dose, take it as soon as you remember, then resume your regular schedule. Do not double-dose.
- Do not stop taking this medication without consulting your doctor.
- Drink lots of fluids (2-3 liters/day) unless on a fluid-restricted diet.
- Use caution when driving or performing tasks where alertness is needed, until you know how this medication affects you.
- Do not take any new medications, including over-the-counter medications, while taking uric aid-lowering prescriptions without talking to a doctor first.
- You may experience temporary hair loss while on this medication.
- It may take six to 12 months of treatment to get the full benefits in preventing gout attacks.

Side Effects:
- Drowsiness
- Nausea
- Vomiting
- Heartburn

Allopurinol can, in rare cases, cause potentially fatal side effects. Contact your doctor *immediately* if you have any of these side effects:
- Skin rash or lesions
- Painful urination
- Blood in your urine or stool
- Unresolved nausea or vomiting
- Numbness of the extremities
- Pain or irritation of the eyes
- Swelling of the lips, mouth or tongue
- Unusual fatigue
- Easy bruising or bleeding
- Yellowing of the skin or eyes
- Change in the color of your urine or stool

Probenecid

Uses: Used to treat gout by lowering uric acid levels. Probenecid is a uricosuric drug that increases kidney output of uric acid by helping to prevent uric acid reabsorbtion.

Trade names include: Benemid®, Probalan®, Benuryl®

Tell you doctor if any of these apply to you *before* taking this medication:
- If you have a blood disorder or disease
- If you have kidney disease or have ever had kidney stones
- If you recently had radiation therapy
- If you have stomach ulcers
- If you have ever had an unusual or allergic reaction to probenecid, other medicines, foods, dyes or preservatives
- If you are pregnant or trying to get pregnant
- If you are breast-feeding

Drugs and herbal products that can interact with probenecid:
- Alcohol
- Allopurinol
- Anti-inflammatory drugs, including indomethacin and naproxen
- Antibiotics such as penicillin
- Antibiotics based on sulfonamides (known as sulfa drugs)
- Antiviral medicines such as acyclovir, famciclovir, ganciclovir
- Aspirin and aspirin-containing medicines
- Barbiturates
- Benzodiazepine-based drugs such as Valium and Xanax
- Clofibrate
- Dapsone
- Diazoxide
- Dyphylline
- Entacapone
- Ethambutol
- Heparin
- Lorazepam
- Mecamylamine
- Methotrexate
- Nitrofurantoin

Probenecid _____

- Pyrazinamide (PZA)
- Rifampin
- Water pills (diuretics)
- Zidovudine

Other Information:

- Take as prescribed. If you miss a dose, take it as soon as you remember, then resume your regular schedule. Do not double-dose.
- Do not stop taking this medication without consulting your doctor.
- Drink lots of fluids (2-3 liters/day) unless on a fluid-restricted diet.
- Aspirin or aspirin-containing medications can reduce the effectiveness of this medication.
- Taking NSAIDs with this medication will increase the potency of the NSAIDs. Discuss with your doctor how this affects the dose of NSAIDs used for acute gout attacks.
- Take with food, antacids or milk to reduce the chance of gastrointestinal problems.
- If you are diabetic, you will need to use serum glucose monitoring.
- Use caution when driving or performing tasks where alertness is needed until you know how this medication affects you.
- It may take 6-12 months of treatment to get the full benefits in preventing gout attacks.
- A formulation of probenecid exists that also contains 0.5 mg of colchicine. This medication is useful when colchicine prophylaxis is used.

Side Effects:

- Dizziness
- Lightheadedness
- Nervousness
- Nausea
- Vomiting
- Headache
- Indigestion
- Loss of appetite

Probenecid

Contact your doctor *immediately* if you have any of these side effects:
- Skin rash or itching
- Persistent headache
- Blood in the urine or painful urination
- Excessive tiredness
- Easy bruising or bleeding
- Sore gums

Sulfinpyrazone

Uses: Used to treat gout by lowering uric acid levels. Sulfinpyrazone is a uricosuric drug that increases kidney output of uric acid by helping to prevent uric acid reabsorbtion.

Trade names include: Anturane®, Anturan®

Tell you doctor if any of these apply to you *before* taking this medication:
- If you have blood disorders or disease
- If you have liver disease
- If you have kidney disease or kidney stones
- If you have recently had chemotherapy or radiation therapy
- If you have stomach ulcers
- If you have ever had an unusual reaction to sulfinpyrazone, salicylates such as aspirin, phenylbutazone, non-steroidal anti-inflammatory drugs (NSAIDs) such as ibuprofen, other medicines, foods, dyes or preservatives
- If you are pregnant or trying to get pregnant
- If you are breast-feeding

What drugs and herbal products that can interact with sulfinpyrazone:
- Acetaminophen or products that contain acetaminophen (such as Tylenol)
- Anti-inflammatory medications such as NSAIDs
- Aspirin and aspirin-containing medicines
- Niacin

- Theophylline
- Tolbutamide
- Verapamil
- Warfarin

Other Information:
- Use exactly as prescribed.
- Taking with food and a full glass of water reduces the chance of gastro-intestinal problems.
- Do not drink alcohol, take aspirin or aspirin-containing medications, acetaminophen or products that contain acetaminophen.
- It is important to drink lots of fluids (2-3 liters/day) to avoid kidney damage, unless you have been instructed to restrict your fluid intake.

Side Effects:
- Nausea
- Vomiting

Contact your doctor *immediately* if you have any of these side effects:
- Skin rash
- Persistent stomach pain
- Painful urination or bloody urine
- Unusual bruising or bleeding
- Fatigue
- Yellowing of eyes and skin

Other Uric Acid Lowering Medications

The following medications are not widely available and/or are in late-stage clinical research drug trials. They may be an option for patients who cannot take any other uric acid-lowering medications. Sign up for a free "beating gout" newsletter at http://www.beatinggout.com/ to stay up to date on the latest developments on gout and gout treatment.

Oxipurinol – When allopurinol enters the body it is quickly broken down into oxipurinol. It is oxipurinol that actually inhibits uric acid production in the body. About 50% of people who have dangerous reactions to allopurinol tolerate oxipurinol well. However, about 30% have the same reactions they did on allopurinol--therefore it should be tried with extreme caution on people who have had severe reactions to allopurinol.[4] Unfortunately, oxipurinol is not widely available and can only be ordered directly from the manufacturer in small quantities.[9,43] However, if you have very high uric acid levels, have reactions to allopurinol and cannot take any of the other uric acid-lowering drugs, it would be worth discussing with your doctor.

Febuxostat – Febuxostat is a new xanthine oxidase inhibitor drug like allopurinol that is currently in stage three drug trials (the last stage prior to release). Current tests show that febuxostat is more effective than allopurinol and has fewer side effects.[9] Also, the chemistry of febuxostat is significantly different than allopurinol, which means that there is a good chance that people who have adverse reactions to allopurinol will not have the same reactions to febuxostat. Febuxostat is removed from the body by the liver, making it an excellent drug for patients with kidney problems.[7,19] If approved, this would make febuxostat the first major uric acid-lowering drug to come on the market in more than 40 years.

Puricase – As mentioned in Chapter One, all animals except apes and humans produce an enzyme called uricase, which breaks down uric acid and removes it from the body. Puricase is a drug which takes this enzyme and modifies it to make it more compatible with human biology. As of the printing of this book, it has completed phase three clinical trials, and the manufacturer will likely soon apply to the FDA for approval. If approved, this drug should be available on the market sometime in 2009. Puricase is considered a "last resort" drug and will likely only be given to patients who cannot take any other uric acid-lowering medication. Also, it is an injection-only drug, making it more difficult to administer. The dose is given as an injection in the arm once every two to four weeks. About 25% of patients have reported mild to moderate side effects as a result of the injections.[128]

Appendix C: More Information For Doctors

Below is a list of excellent articles on gout management and treatments:

Zhang W, Doherty M, Pascual E, *et al.* EULAR evidence based recommendations for gout. Part I: Diagnosis. Report of a task force of the standing committee for international clinical studies including therapeutics (ESCISIT). Annals of Rheumatic Disease. 2006;65:1301-1311.

Zhang W, Doherty M, Bardin T, *et al.* EULAR evidence based recommendations for gout. Part II: Management. Report of a task force of the EULAR Standing Committee For International Clinical Studies Including Therapeutics (ESCISIT). Annals of Rheumatic Disease. 2006;65;1312-1324.

Nuki G. Gout. Medicine. 2006;34(10):417-423.

Wortmann RL. Recent advances in the management of gout and hyperuricemia. Current Opinion in Rheumatology. 2005;17:319-324.

Choi HK, *et al.* Pathogenesis of Gout. Annals of Internal Medicine. 2005;143:499-516.

Schlesinger N, Management of Acute and Chronic Gouty Arthritis. Drugs. 2004;64(21):2399-2416.

Keith MP, Gilliland WR. Updates in the Management of Gout. The American Journal of Medicine 2007;120:221-224.

Interesting articles on hyperuricemia and its co-morbidities:

Becker MA, Jolly M. Hyperuricemia and Associated Diseases. Rheumatic Disease Clinics of North America. 2006;32:275-293.

Vázquez-Mellado J, Hernández EA, Burgos-Vargas R. Primary Prevention in Rheumatology: The Importance of Hyperuricemia. Best Practice & Research Clinical Rheumatology. 2004;18(2):111-124.

Choi HK, Ford ES, *et al.* Prevalence of the Metabolic Syndrome in Patients With Gout: The Third National Health and Nutrition Examination Survey. Arthritis & Rheumatism. 2007;57(1):109-115.

Glossary:

24-hour uric acid test: A medical test in which urine is collected for 24 hours. It is then measured to determine the amount of uric acid removed from the body by the kidneys each day.

Acidic: A characteristic of a substance that is defined by its ability to neutralize alkalis, dissolve some metals and is a corrosive substance, with a pH value below 7.

ACTH: Adrenocorticotropic hormone is a hormone produced and secreted by the pituitary gland. It is available as a medication under the name cosyntropin (Trade name: Cortrosyn®) and synacthen® (synthetic ACTH).

Acute gouty arthritis: Sudden-onset arthritis that is caused by uric acid crystals in the affected joint(s).

Acute myocardial infarction: Commonly called a "heart attack," it is caused by the sudden interruption of blood supply to the heart muscle.

Atkin's™ diet: A program that claims one can lose weight by eliminating carbohydrates from the diet.

Advanced gout: The result of years of untreated gout, characterized by significant joint damage, constant pain and, usually, large tophi.

Alkaline: A characteristic of a substance that is defined by its ability to neutralize acids, dissolve some metals and is a corrosive substance, having a pH value above 7.

Amino Acids: Amino acids occur naturally in plant and animal tissues and are the basic "building blocks" of proteins.

Arthritis: A group of conditions involving damage to the joints of the body.

Ascorbic Acid: Vitamin C.

Asymmetric: Lacking symmetry. Uneven, irregular.

Asymptomatic: Producing or showing no symptoms.

Atherosclerotic: A condition in which the blood vessels are inflamed and/or obstructed.

Benzbromarone: A powerful uricosuric drug removed from the market in many countries, including the US, due to reports of fatal liver failure.

Blood pressure: the force exerted by circulating blood on the walls of blood vessels. Consisting of two values, the systolic arterial pressure (the top number) is defined as the peak pressure in the arteries; the diastolic arterial pressure (the bottom number) is the lowest pressure. The optimal adult blood pressure is 120/80.

BMI: Body Mass Index is a weight-to-height ratio calculated by dividing a person's weight in kilograms by the square of his height in meters. A BMI of 18.5-25 is considered healthy; 25-30 is overweight; over 30 is obese; and over 40 is morbidly obese. Below 18.5 is considered underweight and is also considered unhealthy.

Bromelain: An enzyme found in some fruits, such as pineapples.

Burdock Root: Roots from one of a group of trees called biennial thistles.

Cardiovascular disease (CVD): A class of diseases that involve the heart or blood vessels.

Chronic: Persisting for a long time or constantly reoccurring.

Colchicine: A drug made from the autumn crocus or meadow saffron flower (Colchicum autumnale) and used to treat gout.

Coronary bypass: Surgery to restore blood flow to the heart muscle after it has been obstructed by atherosclerotic narrowing.

Coronary heart disease (CHD): Also called coronary artery disease (CAD), this refers to a condition that obstructs the arteries of the heart.

Corticosteroids: A class of steroid hormones that are produced in the adrenal gland. Glucocorticoids are used in gout treatment and work by controlling inflammation.

COX-2 Inhibitors: A form of non-steroidal anti-inflammatory drug (NSAID) that directly targets COX-2, an enzyme responsible for inflammation and pain. COX-2 inhibitors typically have a lower risk of gastrointestinal bleeding when compared to other NSAIDs.

Crystallize: To change from a liquid state to a solid state while forming crystals.

Crystal-related arthropathy: A more technical term for arthritis caused by crystals.

CT scan: Stands for computed tomography. Uses computer imaging to generate three-dimensional images from X-rays.

Culture (Bacterial): The cultivation of bacteria in an artificial medium containing nutrients.

Desensitize: To expose someone to increasingly larger doses of a substance that they are sensitive to until the body becomes tolerant of it.

Devil's Claw: Also called grapple plant or wood spider. Devil's Claw is believed to have analgesic, sedative and diuretic properties.

Diuretics: Includes any drug that elevates the body's rate of urine excretion.

Dyslipidemia: A disruption in the amount of lipids in the blood.

Enzyme: Proteins that catalyze (accelerate) chemical reactions.

Fasting: Abstaining from some or all kinds of food or drink.

First metatarsophalangeal joint: Second joint of the big toe from the tip.

Folic acid: Vitamin B9, also known as folate.

Fructose: A simple reducing sugar found in many foods. It is one of the three most important blood sugars, along with glucose and galactose.

Helix of the ear: The outer rim of the ear.

Hepatitis: Injury to the liver characterized by the presence of inflammatory cells in the liver tissue. This term can be use to describe any type of injury to the liver, including injury due to drug allergies, drug interactions or more commonly, injury due to viral or bacterial disease.

Hepatic: Referring to the liver.

High-fat dairy: Any dairy product that is not a low- or reduced-fat variety.

High-resolution ultrasound: Non-invasive medical imaging devices that use sound waves to generate highly detailed images of the inside of living beings.

Homeopathic therapies: Treatment using a substance that can produce, in a healthy person, symptoms similar to those of the illness. The substance is diluted to the point where it is unlikely that any of the original substance remains in the remedy. For example, a 6C dilution results in one part of the original substance in 1,000,000,000,000 (1 trillion) parts of water.

Hyperlipidaemia: Excessive lipids (fats) in the blood

Hypertriglyceridaemia: excessive triglycerides in the blood.

Hyperuricemia: Excessive uric acid in the blood.

Idiopathic: Of unknown cause.

Immune system: The body's system to fight infection and disease.

Inflammation: The biological response of blood vessel tissue to harmful stimuli, such as pathogens, damaged cells or irritants. It is a protective attempt by the body to remove the injurious stimuli, as well as initiate the healing process.

Insulin resistance: A condition in which normal amounts of insulin are inadequate to produce a normal insulin response from fat, muscle and liver cells. It is often the result of a high-carbohydrate diet.

Intercritical periods: The period in between acute gout attacks.

Intra-articular: Within the joint.

Intra-muscular: Within the muscle.

IV (Intravenous): Within the vein or medication infused directly into the vein.

Ketosis: A metabolic stage occurring when the liver converts fat into fatty acids and ketone bodies, which can then be used by the body for energy.

Kidney stones: Crystals of various chemicals excreted by the kidneys, most commonly uric acid. These crystals form in the kidneys and impair kidney function, as well as cause severe pain.

Lipoprotein (High/low density): A biochemical assembly that contains both proteins and lipids. Used by the body to transport fats.

Losartan (Cozaar®): A high blood pressure medication that can also lower uric acid levels by increasing excretion.

Low-fat dairy: Reduced-fat dairy products, including skim milk.

Metabolic syndrome: A collection of conditions that result in an increased likelihood of cardiovascular disease and heart attacks, diabetes, stroke and numerous types of cancer.

Metabolization: A set of chemical reactions that occur in living organisms in order to maintain life.

mg/dL: A unit of measure commonly used in the United States in medical applications. Refers to milligrams per deciliter (100 milliliters).

Micronisedfenofibrate (Tricor®): A cholesterol-lowering medication that also lowers uric acid levels by increasing excretion.

MRI (magnetic resonance imaging): Uses high-power magnetic fields and radio waves to non-invasively image the inside of living bodies.

Mutation: A random change in the genes that make up an organism. Can be the result of a copying error or caused by external influences such as radiation.

Necrosis: The technical name for the death of cells or tissue.

Niacin: Nicotinic acid, more commonly known as vitamin B3. Niacin can raise uric acid levels.

NSAIDs: Short for non-steroidal anti-inflammatory drugs. These drugs work by inhibiting the body's ability to cause inflammation.

Nuclear medicine (bone scans): A test used to visually detect bone abnormalities.

Obesity: Excessively fat or overweight. Defined as a Body Mass Index above 30.

Omega-3 fatty acids: A family of polyunsaturated fatty acids found to have many positive health benefits.

Orally: Taken through the mouth.

Over-produce: To create too much of something.

Peptic ulcer: An ulcer (either sore or weakness) of the gastrointestinal tract, including the mouth, esophagus, stomach and intestines.

pH: A measure of the acidity or alkalinity of a solution. The pH scale ranges from 0 to 14, with 0 being most acidic, 14 being the most alkaline, and 7 being neutral.

Piroxicam: A non-steroidal anti-inflammatory drug that is available in prescription strength only.

Podagra: Refers to gout of the big toe. From the Greek words "pous," or "pod" meaning "foot" and "agra," meaning "seizure."

Primary gout: Gout that is not caused by an underlying medical condition.

Probenecid: A medication used to treat gout by preventing the reabsorbtion of uric acid in the kidneys.

Prophylaxis: Action taken to prevent disease by specified means or against a specific disease.

Protein: Any of a class of organic compounds that consist of large molecules, composed of one or more long chains of amino acids, which are an essential part of all living organisms. They are structural components of body tissues such as muscle, hair, collagen, etc., and of enzymes and antibodies. Proteins are also referred to as a component of food.

Pseudogout: A form of arthritis that causes symptoms similar to gout, but is caused by calcium pyrophosphate crystals rather than uric acid crystals.

Purines: A class of chemicals with a double-ring structure. Purines are the chemicals that the body metabolizes into uric acid.

Renal: Relating to the kidneys.

Rheumatoid arthritis: A chronic, inflammatory autoimmune disorder that causes the immune system to attack the joints.

Secondary gout: Gout caused by an underlying medical condition.

Sensitivity: With medication, this refers to the degree to which a patient has adverse reactions.

Septic: Infected with bacteria or fungus.

Serum uric acid: The quantity of uric acid in blood serum (the liquid part of blood).

Stroke: Damage or death of brain tissue caused by bleeding or the obstruction of blood vessels (causing oxygen starvation).

Super-saturation: To increase the concentration of a solution beyond the normal saturation point.

Synovial fluid: Fluid from inside a joint.

Tophi (pl. tophus): Collections of uric acid that can form anywhere in the body, but are most common around the joints of the hands and feet, as well as the helix of the ears. Latin for "stone."

Toxemia of pregnancy (pre-eclampsia): A medical condition in which hypertension arises during pregnancy (pregnancy-induced hypertension) in association with significant amounts of protein in the urine.

Toxicity: Referring to how poisonous a substance is.

Type-2 diabetes: A metabolic disorder that is primarily characterized by insulin resistance, relative insulin deficiency and hyperglycemia.

Ulcerate: To develop into or become affected by an ulcer.

Under-excrete: To remove from the body too slowly, usually though the urine.

Urate: Refers to the salt of uric acid (monosodium uric acid), but is commonly used interchangeably with uric acid. In this book, urate refers to uric acid in a crystal state.

Uric acid: A chemical classified as a purine that is a major cause of gout.

Uricase: An enzyme found in all mammals except apes and man that breaks down uric acid into a chemical more easily removed from the body.

Uricosuric drugs: Drugs that increase the excretion of uric acid through the kidneys.

White blood cells: Immune system cells (also known as leukocytes), which defend the body against both infectious disease and foreign materials.

Xanthine oxidase inhibitor drugs: Drugs that block one of the chemical processes in the body that creates uric acid.

μmol/L: A unit of measure used in many parts of the world for medical applications. Refers to micromoles per liter.

References:

1. Keith MP, Gilliland WR, Updates in the Management of Gout. The American Journal of Medicine. 2007;120:221-224.

2. McGill NW, Gout and other crystal-associated arthropathies. Bailliére's Clinical Rheumatology. 2000;14(3):445-460.

3. Pascual E, Sivera F, Why is gout so poorly managed? Annals of Rheumatic Disease. 2007;66;1269-1270.

4. Nuki G, Gout. Medicine. 2006;34(10):417-423.

5. Singh J, *et al.* Quality of Care for Gout in the US Needs Improvement. Arthritis & Rheumatism. 2007;57(5):822-829.

6. Vázquez-Mellado J, Hernández EA, Burgos-Vargas R., Primary Prevention in Rheumatology: The Importance of Hyperuricemia. Best Practice & Research Clinical Rheumatology. 2004;18(2):111–124.

7. Eggebeen A, Gout: An Update. American Family Physician. 2007;76(6):801-808.

8. Smelser CD, *et al.* Gout. eMedicine. Sept. 25, 2005.

9. Schlesinger N, Management of Acute and Chronic Gouty Arthritis. Drugs. 2004;64(21):2399-2416.

10. Altera N, Vaturi M, *et al.* Effect of Weather Conditions on Acute Gouty Arthritis. Journal of Rheumatology. 1994;23(1):22-24.

11. Robins, K. Basic Pathology. W. B. Saunders Company (1987);98-102.

12. Wortmann, R, Effective management of Gout [Editorial reply]. The American Journal of Medicine. 1999;107:406.

13. Chen XL, Schumacher HR, Gout: can we create an evidence-based systematic approach to diagnosis and management? Best Practice & Research Clinical Rheumatology. 2006;20(4):673-684.

14. Weaver AL, Case 3: Acute Gout – Risk Factors and Inappropriate Therapy. American Journal of Medicine. 2006;119(11A):S9–S12.

15. Yokam T, Rowe L, Essentials of Skeletal Radiology. Williams and Wilkins (1987);659-665.

16. Bhandaru R, Acharya R, *et al.* Poster presented at the ACR Meeting 2007: Prevalence of Spinal Gout. Number1602, Poster Board Number 273.

17. Berger JS, *et al.* Gout-Induced Arthropathy in a Knee Following Total Arthroplasty: A Case Report. Archives of Physical Medicine and Rehabilitation. 2007;88.

18. Zhang W, Doherty M, Pascual E, *et al.* EULAR evidence based recommendations for gout. Part I: Diagnosis. Report of a task force of the standing committee for international clinical studies including therapeutics (ESCISIT). Annals of Rheumatic Disease. 2006;65:1301–1311.

19. Wortmann RL, Recent advances in the management of gout and hyperuricemia. Current Opinion in Rheumatology. 2005;17:319-324.

20. Osterhaus, *et al.* Poster presented at the ACR Meeting 2005. San Diego, CA.

21. Roddy, E., Zhang, W., Doherty, M., Is gout associated with reduced quality of life? A case-control study. Rheumatology. 2007;46:1441–1444.

22. Kleinman, *et al.* Poster presented at the ACR Meeting 2005. San Diego, CA.

References

23. Klippel JH. Primer on the Rheumatic Diseases, Edition 12. Atlanta: Arthritis Foundation. 2001. Page 313.

24. Falasca GF. Metabolic diseases: gout. Clinics in Dermatology. 2006;24:498-508.

25. Wortmann R. Effective Management of Gout: An Analogy. The American Journal of Medicine. 1998;105:513-514.

26. Jordan KM, Cameron JS, et al. British Society for Rheumatology and British Health Professionals in Rheumatology Guideline for the Management of Gout. Rheumatology. 2007;46:1372-1374.

27. Zhang W, Doherty M, Bardin T, et al. EULAR evidence based recommendations for gout. Part II: Management. Report of a task force of the EULAR Standing Committee For International Clinical Studies Including Therapeutics (ESCISIT). Annals of Rheumatic Disease. 2006;65;1312-1324.

28. Schumacher HR, et al. Randomised double blind trial of etoricoxib and indometacin in treatment of acute gouty arthritis. British Medical Journal. 2002 324: 1488-1492.

29. Rubin BR. Efficacy and safety profile of treatment with etoricoxib 120 mg once daily compared with indomethacin 50 mg three times daily in acute gout. Arthritis & Rheumatism. 2004;50:598-606.

30. Pleuvry BJ. Drugs used to treat muscle and joint disease. Anesthesia and Intensive Care Medicine. 2006;7(3):104-106.

31. Weinstein J. Effective treatment of Gout [Letter to the Editor]. American Journal of Medicine 1999;107:406.

32. Terkeltaub RA. Gout. The New England Journal of Medicine. 2003;349:1647-1655.

33. Wright JD, Pinto AB. Clinical Manifestations and Treatment of Gout. Primary Care Update for Ob/Gyns. 2003;10(1):19-23.

34. Alldred A. Gout – pharmacological management. Hospital Pharmacist. 2005;12:395-400.

35. Baxter K, et al. Stockley's Drug Interactions. Eighth Edition. Chicago:Pharmaceutical Press.

36. http://www.fda.gov/cder/drug/infopage/COX2/NSAIDmedguide.pdf accessed 2/19/2008.

37. Karalliedde L, Henry AJ. (1998) Handbook of Drug Interactions. New York:Arnold.

38. Niel E, Scherrmann JM. Colchicine today. Joint Bone Spine. 2006;73:672-678.

39. Aherin MJ, et al. Does colchicine work? Australia and New Zealand Journal of Medicine. 1987;17:301-304.

40. Varughese GI, et al. A Caveat in the Management of Acute Gout – Letter to the editor. The American Journal of Medicine. 2007;120:e31.

41. Hough DW. Gouty Arthritis: The Missed Diagnosis. Dynamic Chiropractic. 2000;18(20).

42. Annemans L, Spaepen E, et al. Gout in the UK and Germany: prevalence, comorbidities and management in general practice 2000-2005. Annals of Rheumatic Disease. Published online: Nov 2, 2007.

43. Bardin T. Current management of gout in patients unresponsive or allergic to allopurinol. Joint Bone Spine. 2004;71:481-485.

44. Shekarriz B, Stoller M. Uric acid nephrolithiasis: current concepts and controversies. Journal of Urology. 2002;168:1307-1314.

45. Choi HK, et al. Pathogenesis of Gout. Annals of Internal Medicine. 2005;143:499-516.

46. Perez-Ruiz F, Martin I, Canteli B. Ultrasonographic measurement of tophi as an outcome measure for chronic gout. Journal of Rheumatology. 2007;34(9):1888-93.

47. Perez-Ruiz F, Calabozo M, *et al.* Renal Underexcretion of Uric Acid Is Present in Patients With Apparent High Urinary Uric Acid Output. Arthritis & Rheumatism. 2002;47(6):610-613.

48. Feher MD, Hepburn AL, *et al.* Fenofibrate lowers serum urate in patients treated with allopurinol. Rheumatology. 2003;42:321-325.

49. Finley, MJ. Case 8: Initiation of Urate-Lowering Therapy for Standard Advanced Gout. American Journal of Medicine. 2006;119(11A):S25-S28.

50. Perez-Ruiz, F, *et al.* Effect of Urate-Lowering Therapy on the Velocity of Size Reduction of Tophi in Chronic Gout. Arthritis & Rheumatism. 2002;47(4):356-360.

51. Segal JB, Albert D. Diagnosis of Crystal-Induced Arthritis by Synovial Fluid Examination for Crystals: Lessons from an Imperfect Test. Arthritis Care and Research. 1999;12(6):376-380.

52. Pascual, *et al.* Best Practice and Research in Clinical Rheumatology. 2004;50:2400-2414.

53. Wallace SL, Robinson H, *et al.* Preliminary criteria for the classification of the acute arthritis of primary gout. Arthritis & Rheumatology. 1977;20:896.

54. Coakley G, Mathews C, *et al.* BSR & BHPR, BOA, RCGP and BSAC guidelines for management of the hot swollen joint in adults. Rheumatology. 2006;45:1039-1041.

55. Perez-Ruiz F, Naredo E. Imaging modalities and monitoring measures of gout. Current Opinion in Rheumatology 2007;19:128-133.

56. Coombs RJ, Pinsky ST, Padanilam TG. Bone scan findings of combined gout and septic arthritis in the same digit. Clinical Nuclear Medicine. 2001;26(5):442-443.

57. Haddad RH, Allegra EC. Closer Look At Musculoskeletal Ultrasound. Arthritis Practitioner. 2006;2(3):28-32.

58. Thiele RG, Schlesinger N. Diagnosis of gout by ultrasound. Rheumatology. 2007;46(7):1116-1121.

59. Wright SA, *et al.* High-resolution ultrasonography of the 1st metatarsal phalangeal joint in gout: A controlled study. Annals of the Rheumatic Diseases. 2007;66:859-864.

60. Tavaras JM, Ferrucci JT Jr, editors. Radiology: Diagnosis, Imaging, Intervention. Philadelphia, Pa: JB Lippincott Co; 1993.

61. Velilla-Moliner J, *et al.* Podagra, is it always gout? American Journal of Emergency Medicine. 2004;22(4):320-321.

62. http://www.medicinenet.com/hydroxyapatite/article.htm Accessed: 12/27/07

63. Shmerling RH, Delbanco TL. The rheumatoid factor: an analysis of clinical utility. American Journal of Medicine. 1991;91:528-534.

64. Edwards NL. Case 7: Differential Diagnosis of Advanced Gout. American Journal of Medicine. 2006;119(11A):S23-S24.

65. Kim KY, *et al.* A literature review of the epidemiology and treatment of acute gout. Clinical Therapeutics. 2003;25(6):1617.

66. Choi HK, Atkinson K, Karlson EW, Curhan G. Obesity, weight change, hypertension, diuretic use, and risk of gout in men. Archives of Internal Medicine. 2005;165:742-748.

67. Campion EW, Glynn RJ, DeLabry LO. Asymptomatic hyperuricemia: risks and consequences in the Normative Aging Study. American Journal of Medicine. 1987;82:421-426.

References

68. Roubenoff R. Gout and hyperuricemia. Rheumatic Disease Clinics of North America. 1990;16:539-550.

69. Chen SY, *et al.* Clinical features of familial gout and effects of probable genetic association between gout and its related disorders. Metabolism. 2001;50(10):1203-1207.

70. Bieber JD, Terkeltaub RA, *et al.* Gout: On the Brink of Novel Therapeutic Options for an Ancient Disease. Arthritis & Rheumatism. 2004;50(8):2400-2414.

71. Darmawan J, Lutalo SL. Gout and hyperuricaemia. Bailliére's Clinical Rheumatology. 1995;9(1):83-94.

72. Hasday J, Grum C. Nocturnal Increase of Uricary Uric Acid: Creatinine Ratio. American Review of Respiratory Disease. 1987;135:534-538.

73. Bengmark S. Acute and "chronic" phase reaction—a mother of disease. Clinical Nutrition. 2004;23:1256-1266.

74. McLachlan A, *et al.* Team-based Approach to Assessing and Managing CVD Risk in Gout Patients Using Acute Predict Electronic Clinical Decision Support. Heart, Lung and Circulation. 2007;16:S184.

75. Choi HK, Ford ES, *et al.* Prevalence of the Metabolic Syndrome in Patients With Gout: The Third National Health and Nutrition Examination Survey. Arthritis & Rheumatism. 2007;57(1):109-115.

76. Expert Panel on Detection, Evaluation, and Treatment of High Blood Cholesterol in Adults. Executive Summary of the Third Report of the National Cholesterol Education Program (NCEP) Expert Panel on Detection, Evaluation, and Treatment of High Blood Cholesterol in Adults (Adult Treatment Panel III). Journal of the American Medical Association. 2001;285:2486-2497.

77. Grundy SM. A Constellation of Complications: The Metabolic Syndrome. Clinical Cornerstone. 2005;7(2/3):36-45.

78. Becker MA, Jolly M. Hyperuricemia and Associated Diseases. Rheumatic Disease Clinics of North America. 2006;32:275-293.

79. Niskanen KL, Laaksonen ED, *et al.* Uric Acid Level as a Risk Factor for Cardiovascular and All-Cause Mortality in Middle-aged Men: A Prospective Cohort Study. Archives of Internal Medicine. 2004;164(14):1546-1551.

80. Takahashi S, Moriwaki Y, *et al.* Increased visceral fat accumulation further aggravates the risk of insulin resistance in Gout. Metabolism. 2001;50(4):393-398.

81. Gavin AR, Struthers AD. Hyperuricemia and Adverse Outcomes in Cardiovascular Disease. American Journal of Cardiovascular Drugs. 2003;3(5):309-314.

82. Krishnan E, Baker JF. Gout and the Risk of Acute Myocardial Infarction. Arthritis & Rheumatism. 2006;54(8):2688-2696.

83. Tomita M, *et al.* Does Hyperuricemia affect mortality? A Prospective Cohort Study of Japanese Male Workers. Journal of Epidemiology. 2000;10:403-409.

84. Kang DK, Nakagawa T. Uric acid and chronic renal disease: Possible implication of hyperuricemia on progression of renal disease. Seminars in Nephrology. 2005;25(1):43-49.

85. Tarng DC, *et al.* Renal function in gout patients. American Journal of Nephrology. 1995;15(1):31-7.

86. McCarty CA, *et al.* The Epidemiology of Cataract in Australia. American Journal of Ophthalmology. 1999;128(4):446-465.

87. Harrold LR, Yood RA, *et al.* Sex differences in gout epidemiology: evaluation and treatment. Annals of Rheumatic Disease. 2006;65;1368-1372.

88. Cleland LG, Hill CL, James MJ. Diet and arthritis. Bailliére's Clinical Rheumatology. 1995;9(5):771-785.

89. Pi-Sunyer FX. A Review of Long-Term Studies Evaluating the Efficacy of Weight Loss in Ameliorating Disorders Associated with Obesity. Clinical Therapeutics. 1996;18(6):1006-1035.

90. Gibson T, Rodgers AV, *et al.* A controlled study of diet in patients with gout. Annals of Rheumatic Disease. 1983;42:123-127.

91. Mikuls TR, MacLean CH, *et al.* Quality of care indicators for gout management. Arthritis & Rheumatism. 2004;50(3):937-943.

92. Dessein PH, Shipton EA, *et al.* Beneficial effects of weight loss associated with moderate calorie/carbohydrate restriction, and increased proportional intake of protein and unsaturated fat on serum urate and lipoprotein levels in gout: a pilot study. Annals of Rheumatic Disease. 2000;59;539-543.

93. Eastmond CJ, Garton M, Robins S, Riddoch S. The effects of alcoholic beverages on urate metabolism in gout sufferers. British Journal of Rheumatology. 1995; 34:756-759.

94. Lee SJ, Terkeltaub RA, Kavanaugh A. Recent Developments in Diet and Gout. Current Opinion in Rheumatology. 2006;18(2):193-198.

95. Choi HK, Atkinson K, *et al.* Alcohol intake and risk of incident gout in men: a prospective study. Lancet. 2004;363(9417):1277-1281.

96. Choi HK, Curhan G. Alcohol and Gout (Letter to the Editor). American Journal of Medicine. 2007;120:e5.

97. Kaneko K, Fujimori S, Akaoka I. Changes caused by ethanol intake on metabolism of hypouricemic agents (combination of allopurinol and benzbromarone). Advances in Experimental Medicine and Biology 1991;309A:139-142.

98. Choi HK. Diet, alcohol, and gout: how do we advise patients given recent developments? Current Rheumatology Reports. 2005;7:220-226.

99. Wallace KL, Riedel AA, Joseph-Ridge N, Wortmann R. Increasing prevalence of gout and hyperuricemia over 10 years among older adults in a managed care population. Journal of Rheumatology. 2004;31:1582-1587.

100. Parillo M, Rivellese AA, Ciardullo AV, *et al.* A high-monounsaturated-fat/low-carbohydrate diet improves peripheral insulin sensitivity in non-insulin-dependent diabetic patients. Metabolism. 1992;41:1373-1378.

101. Griffith RW. Diet and gout - a new approach? Health and Age. August 31, 2000.

102. Choi HK, Liu S, Curhan G. Intake of purine-rich foods, protein, and dairy products and relationship to serum levels of uric acid: The Third National Health and Nutrition Examination Survey. Arthritis & Rheumatism. 2005;52(1):283-289.

103. Yu KH, See LC, *et al.* Dietary Factors Associated with Hyperuricemia in Adults. Seminars in Arthritis and Rheumatism. 2007;37(4):243-250.

104. Adapted from: Peckenpaugh NJ. Nutrition Essentials and Diet Therapy: Tenth Edition. St. Louis: Saunders Elsevier, 2007.

105. Hu FB, Rimm E, Smith-Warner SA, *et al.* Reproducibility and validity of dietary patterns assessed with a food frequency questionnaire. American Journal of Clinical Nutrition. 1999;69:243-249.

References

106. Huang HY, Appel LJ, Choi MJ, *et al.* The effects of vitamin C supplementation on serum concentrations of uric acid. Arthritis & Rheumatism. 2005;52:1843-1847.

107. Perez-Ruiz F. New treatments for gout. Joint Bone Spine. 2007;74:313-315.

108. Stein HB, Hasan A, Fox IH. Ascorbic Acid-Induced Uricosuria. Annals of Internal Medicine. 1976;84:385-388.

109. Matzkies F, Berg G, Madl H. The uricosuric action of protein in man. Advances in Experimental Medicine and Biology. 1980;122A:227-231.

110. Lin KC, Lin HY, Chou P. The interaction between uric acid level and other risk factors on the development of gout among asymptomatic hyperuricemia men in a prospective study. Journal of Rheumatology. 2000;27:1501-1505.

111. Schlesinger N, Dietary Factors and Hyperuricaemia. Current Pharmaceutical Design. 2005;11:4133-4138.

112. Murray M, Pizzorno J. Encyclopedia of Natural Medicine. Prima Publishing (1991);332-340.

113. Yamamoto T, Moriwaki Y, *et al.* Effect of sauna bathing and beer ingestion in plasma concentrations of purine bases. Metabolism. 2004;53(6):772-776.

114. Zhang YQ, Chaisson CE, *et al.* Poster presented at the ACR Meeting 2006: High Humidity and High Temperature Increase the Risk of Recurrent Gout Attacks: The Online Case-crossover Gout Study. Number 707, Boston, MA.

115. Gallerani M, Govoni M, *et al.* Seasonal variation in the onset of acute microcrystalline arthritis. Rheumatology. 1999;36:1003-1006.

116. Griffith RW. Gout, or pseudogout? Health and Age. March 12, 2001.

117. Nakagawa T, *et al.* A Causal Role for Uric acid in Fructose-induced Metabolic Syndrome. American Journal of Physiology - Renal Physiology. 2006;290:F625-F631.

118. Choi HK, Curhan G. Coffee, Tea, and Caffeine Consumption and Serum Uric Acid Level: The Third National Health and Nutrition Examination Survey. Arthritis & Rheumatism. 2007;57(5):816-821.

119. Levinson W, *et al.* To Change or Not To Change: "Sounds Like You Have a Dilemma" Annals of Internal Medicine. 2001;135(5):386-391.

120. US Department of Agriculture Food and Nutrition Center. Dietary Reference Intakes for Energy, Carbohydrate. Fiber, Fat, Fatty Acids, Cholesterol, Protein, and Amino Acids (2002/2005).

121. Wantroba AN. Gale Encyclopedia of Alternative Medicine. 2004. Portland:Gale Cengage.

122. Owen PL, Johns T. Xanthine oxidase inhibitory activity of northeastern North American plant remedies used for gout. Journal of Ethnopharmacology. 1999;64:149-160.

123. Jacob R, *et al.* Consumption of Cherries Lowers Plamsa Urate in Healthy Women. Journal of Nutrition. 2003;133(6):1826-1829.

124. Shang A., *et al.* Are the clinical effects of homoeopathy placebo effects? Comparative study of placebo-controlled trials of homoeopathy and allopathy. Lancet. 2005;366:726-732.

125. Vandenbroucke J. P. Homoeopathy and "the growth of truth". Lancet. 2005;366:691-692.

126. Yasgur J. Yasgur's Homeopathic Dictionary and Holistic Health Reference. Fourth Edition. Greenville:Van Hoy Publishers. 1998.

127. All information on indomethacin, naproxen, sulindac, colchicine, allopurinol, probenecid and sulfinpyrazone comes from the following sources unless otherwise noted:

Turkoski BB, *et al.* Drug Information Handbook for Advanced Practice Nursing. Huston, Ohio: Lexi-Comp.

Skidmore-Roth L, *et al.* 2008 Mosby's Nursing Drug Reference. St. Louis: Mosby.

McEvoy GK, *et al.* 2006 AHFS Drug Information. Bathesda: American Society of Health System Pharmacists.

128. http://investor.savient.com/ReleaseDetail.cfm?ReleaseID=291911 accessed on 2/19/08 and http://www.savientpharma.com/pipeline/puricase.asp Accessed on 12/29/07

129. Meigs JB, Wilson PW, Nathan DM, *et al.* Prevalence and characteristics of the metabolic syndromes in the San Antonio Heart and Framingham Offspring Studies. Diabetes. 2003;52:2160-2167.

130. Ford ES, Giles WH, Dietz WH. Prevalence of the metabolic syndrome among US adults. Journal of the American Medical Association. 2002;287:356-359.

131. Perez-Ruiz F, Calabozo M, *et al.* Renal Underexcretion of Uric Acid Is Present in Patients With Apparent High Urinary Uric Acid Output. Arthritis & Rheumatism. 2002;47(6):610-613.

References to claims made on the cover not otherwise discussed in this book:

78% of patients do not receive proper care:

Singh JA, *et al.* Quality of Care for Gout in the US Needs Improvement. Arthritis & Rheumatism. 2007;57(5):833-829.

5.1 million Americans with gout and those with gout miss an average of 4.6 days of work which reduces productivity by 2%.

Kleinman NL, *et al.* The impact of gout on work absence and productivity. Value Health. 2007;10(4):231-237.

Index:

Quick Order Form

Beating Gout makes a great gift! Order a copy today.

Fax Orders: 716-404-2551. Send this form
Online Orders: Visit http://www.beatinggout.com
Postal Orders: Mail this form to:
Make checks payable to "Ayerware Publishing."
Ayerware Publishing
P.O. Box 1098
Williamsville, NY 14231-1098

Please send me _____ copies of Beating Gout at $21.95 (£12.95) each.

Name: _____

Address: _____

City: _____ State: _____ Zip: _____

Telephone: _____

E-mail: _____

Sales Tax: Please add the appropriate sales tax to
orders shipped to New York addresses.
Shipping: Add $5 for 1-2 books,
$10 for 3-10 books and $15 for 10-20 books.
For larger quantities, e-mail: info@ayerware.com
International Shipping: $9 for the first book,
plus $5 for each additional book.

**Visit http://www.ayerware.com/ for a
full listing of products by Ayerware Publishing!**

Quick Order Form

Beating Gout makes a great gift! Order a copy today.

Fax Orders: 716-404-2551. Send this form
Online Orders: Visit http://www.beatinggout.com
Postal Orders: Mail this form to:
Make checks payable to "Ayerware Publishing."
Ayerware Publishing
P.O. Box 1098
Williamsville, NY 14231-1098

Please send me _____ copies of Beating Gout at $21.95 (£12.95) each.

Name: _____

Address: _____

City: _____ State: _____ Zip: _____

Telephone: _____

E-mail: _____

Sales Tax: Please add the appropriate sales tax to
orders shipped to New York addresses.
Shipping: Add $5 for 1-2 books,
$10 for 3-10 books and $15 for 10-20 books.
For larger quantities, e-mail: info@ayerware.com
International Shipping: $9 for the first book,
plus $5 for each additional book.

**Visit http://www.ayerware.com/ for a
full listing of products by Ayerware Publishing!**